A FRAMEWORK FOR
EDUCATING
HEALTH PROFESSIONALS
TO ADDRESS THE
SOCIAL DETERMINANTS
OF HEALTH

Committee on Educating Health Professionals to Address the
Social Determinants of Health

Board on Global Health

Institute of Medicine

The National Academies of
SCIENCES · ENGINEERING · MEDICINE

THE NATIONAL ACADEMIES PRESS
Washington, DC
www.nap.edu

THE NATIONAL ACADEMIES PRESS   500 Fifth Street, NW   Washington, DC 20001

This study was supported by contracts between the National Academy of Sciences and the Academic Collaborative for Integrative Health, the Academy of Nutrition and Dietetics, the Accreditation Council for Graduate Medical Education, the Aetna Foundation, the Alliance for Continuing Education in the Health Professions, the American Academy of Family Physicians, the American Academy of Nursing, the American Association of Colleges of Nursing, the American Association of Colleges of Osteopathic Medicine, the American Association of Colleges of Pharmacy, the American Board of Family Medicine, the American Board of Internal Medicine, the American College of Nurse-Midwives, the American College of Obstetricians and Gynecologists/American Board of Obstetrics and Gynecology, the American Council of Academic Physical Therapy, the American Dental Education Association, the American Medical Association, the American Occupational Therapy Association, the American Psychological Association, the American Society for Nutrition, the American Speech–Language–Hearing Association, the Association of American Medical Colleges, the Association of American Veterinary Medical Colleges, the Association of Schools and Colleges of Optometry, the Association of Schools and Programs of Public Health, the Association of Schools of the Allied Health Professions, the Council of Academic Programs in Communication Sciences and Disorders, the Council on Social Work Education, Ghent University, Health Resources and Services Administration, the Jonas Center for Nursing and Veterans Healthcare, the Josiah Macy Jr. Foundation, Kaiser Permanente, the National Academies of Practice, the National Association of Social Workers, the National Board for Certified Counselors, Inc. and Affiliates, the National Board of Medical Examiners, the National League for Nursing, the Office of Academic Affiliations—Veterans Health Administration, the Organization for Associate Degree Nursing, the Physician Assistant Education Association, the Robert Wood Johnson Foundation, the Society for Simulation in Healthcare, Training for Health Equity Network, the Uniformed Services University of the Health Sciences, and the University of Toronto. Any opinions, findings, conclusions, or recommendations expressed in this publication do not necessarily reflect the views of any organization or agency that provided support for the project.

International Standard Book Number-13:   978-0-309-39262-4
International Standard Book Number-10:   0-309-39262-4
Digital Object Identifier: 10.17226/21923
Library of Congress Control Number: 2016955391

Additional copies of this report are available for sale from the National Academies Press, 500 Fifth Street, NW, Keck 360, Washington, DC 20001; (800) 624-6242 or (202) 334-3313; http://www.nap.edu.

Suggested citation: National Academies of Sciences, Engineering, and Medicine. 2016. *A framework for educating health professionals to address the social determinants of health*. Washington, DC: The National Academies Press. doi: 10.17226/21923.

The National Academies of
SCIENCES · ENGINEERING · MEDICINE

The **National Academy of Sciences** was established in 1863 by an Act of Congress, signed by President Lincoln, as a private, nongovernmental institution to advise the nation on issues related to science and technology. Members are elected by their peers for outstanding contributions to research. Dr. Ralph J. Cicerone is president.

The **National Academy of Engineering** was established in 1964 under the charter of the National Academy of Sciences to bring the practices of engineering to advising the nation. Members are elected by their peers for extraordinary contributions to engineering. Dr. C. D. Mote, Jr., is president.

The **National Academy of Medicine** (formerly the Institute of Medicine) was established in 1970 under the charter of the National Academy of Sciences to advise the nation on medical and health issues. Members are elected by their peers for distinguished contributions to medicine and health. Dr. Victor J. Dzau is president.

The three Academies work together as the **National Academies of Sciences, Engineering, and Medicine** to provide independent, objective analysis and advice to the nation and conduct other activities to solve complex problems and inform public policy decisions. The Academies also encourage education and research, recognize outstanding contributions to knowledge, and increase public understanding in matters of science, engineering, and medicine.

Learn more about the National Academies of Sciences, Engineering, and Medicine at **www.national-academies.org**.

COMMITTEE ON EDUCATING HEALTH PROFSSIONALS TO ADDRESS THE SOCIAL DETERMINANTS OF HEALTH

SANDRA D. LANE (*Chair*), Laura J. and L. Douglas Meredith Professor of Public Health and Anthropology, Syracuse University

JORGE DELVA, Professor and Associate Dean, University of Michigan School of Social Work

JULIAN FISHER, Research Associate, Peter L. Reichertz Institute for Medical Informatics, University of Braunschweig Institute of Technology, and Hannover Medical School

BIANCA FROGNER, Associate Professor and Director, Center for Health Workforce Studies, Department of Family Medicine, University of Washington School of Medicine

CARA V. JAMES, Director, Office of Minority Health, Centers for Medicare & Medicaid Services

MALUAL MABUR, Health Promotion Specialist and Community Health Outreach Worker, City of Portland, Maine; Student, University of New England

LAURA MAGAÑA VALLADARES, Academic Dean, National Institute of Public Health, Mexico

SPERO M. MANSON, Distinguished Professor and Director, Centers for American Indian & Alaska Native Health, University of Colorado Denver

ADEWALE TROUTMAN, Associate Dean for Health Equity and Community Engagement, University of South Florida

ANTONIA M. VILLARRUEL, Professor and Margaret Bond Simon Dean of Nursing, University of Pennsylvania School of Nursing

Consultants

SUSAN SCRIMSHAW, President, The Sage Colleges
SARA WILLEMS, Professor, Inequity in Health Care, Ghent University
KAREN ANDERSON, Senior Program Officer, Institute of Medicine
RONA BRIERE, Consultant Editor

National Academies of Sciences, Engineering, and Medicine Staff

PATRICIA A. CUFF, Senior Program Officer
MEGAN M. PEREZ, Research Associate
BRIDGET CALLAGHAN, Research Assistant

Reviewers

This report has been reviewed in draft form by individuals chosen for their diverse perspectives and technical expertise. The purpose of this independent review is to provide candid and critical comments that will assist the institution in making its published report as sound as possible and to ensure that the report meets institutional standards for objectivity, evidence, and responsiveness to the study charge. The review comments and draft manuscript remain confidential to protect the integrity of the deliberative process. We wish to thank the following individuals for their review of this report:

RAPHAEL BOSTIC, University of Southern California School of Public Policy
ANDREIA BRUNO, International Pharmaceutical Federation
FRANCISCO EDUARDO DE CAMPOS, National Open University for the Unified Health System
FERNANDO A. GUERRA, University of Texas Health Science Center, San Antonio, Texas
CAMARA PHYLLIS JONES, Morehouse School of Medicine
ARTHUR KAUFMAN, University of New Mexico School of Medicine
PAULA LANTZ, University of Michigan School of Public Policy
NANDI A. MARSHALL, Armstrong State University Department of Health Sciences
DAVID T. TAKEUCHI, Boston College School of Social Work

Although the reviewers listed above provided many constructive comments and suggestions, they were not asked to endorse the report's conclusions or recommendations, nor did they see the final draft of the report before its release. The review of this report was overseen by **KATHLEEN DRACUP,** University of California, San Francisco, and **SUSAN J. CURRY,** University of Iowa. They were responsible for making certain that an independent examination of this report was carried out in accordance with institutional procedures and that all review comments were carefully considered. Responsibility for the final content of this report rests entirely with the authoring committee and the institution.

Contents

Boxes and Figures

BOXES

xi

Glossary[1]

Community-based education "consists of learning activities that use the community extensively as a learning environment" (WHO, 1987, p. 8).

Community-engaged learning is an educational process by which people are enabled to become actively and genuinely involved in defining the issues of concern to them; in making decisions about factors that affect their lives; in formulating and implementing policies; in planning, developing and delivering services; and in taking action to active change (adapted from WHO, 2002).

Community Oriented Primary Care integrates clinical medicine with public health at the community level and is directed to the epidemiologically defined health needs of the population under care (TUFH, 2000).

Continuing professional development "aims to enhance knowledge and improve performance leading to quality outcomes" (WHO, 2008a).

Equity is "the absence of avoidable or remediable differences among groups of people, whether those groups are defined socially, economically, demographically, or geographically" (WHO, 2016a).

---

[1] Note that this glossary includes only terms that appear in the report. The committee recognizes that many definitions for these terms exist and that some definitions evolve over time.

Experiential learning involves concrete experiences, reflective observation, abstract conceptualization, and application of knowledge (Kolb, 1984).

Framework is "the ideas, information, and principles that form the structure of an organization or plan" (Cambridge University Press, 2016a).

Health disparities are health outcomes seen to a greater or lesser extent between populations of differing race or ethnicity, sex, sexual identity, age, disability, socioeconomic status, and geographic location (HHS, 2016).

Health impact assessment is a combination of procedures, methods, and tools by which a policy, program, product, or service may be judged concerning its effects on the health of the population (WHO, 1998).

Health in all policies is a policy or reform designed to "secure healthier communities, by integrating public health actions with primary care and by pursuing healthy public policies across sectors" (WHO, 2008b, 2011).

Health inequities "involve more than inequality with respect to health determinants, access to the resources needed to improve and maintain health or health outcomes. They also entail a failure to avoid or overcome inequalities that infringe on fairness and human rights norms" (WHO, 2016a).

Health professionals "are the service providers who link people to technology, information, and knowledge. They are also caregivers, communicators and educators, team members, managers, leaders, and policy makers" (Frenk et al., 2010).

Interprofessional education "occurs when two or more professions learn about, from and with each other to enable effective collaboration and improve health outcomes" (WHO, 2010).

Lifelong learning is a continuum of learning throughout the life course aimed at "improving knowledge, skills, and competences within a personal, civic, social, and/or employment-related perspective" (The Council of the European Union, 2002).

Model is "something built or drawn especially to show how something much larger would look" (Cambridge University Press, 2016b).

Problem-based learning is a way of delivering a curriculum in order to develop problem solving skills as well as assisting learners with the acquisition of necessary knowledge and skills. Students work cooperatively in groups to seek solutions to real-world problems, set to engage students' curiosity and initiate learning the subject matter (WHO, 2008a).

Social determinants of health are "the conditions in which people are born, grow, live, work, and age, including the health system. These circumstances are shaped by the distribution of money, power, and resources at global, national, and local levels, which are themselves influenced by policy choices. The social determinates of health are mostly responsible for health inequities—the unfair and avoidable differences in health status seen within and between countries" (WHO, 2016b).

Transformative learning is education that emphasizes searching, analysis, and synthesis of information for decision making; achieving core competencies for effective teamwork in health systems; and creative adaptation of global resources to address local priorities (Frenk et al., 2010).

REFERENCES

Cambridge University Press. 2016a. *Framework.* http://dictionary.cambridge.org/us/dictionary/english/framework (accessed February 2, 2016).

Cambridge University Press. 2016b. *Model.* http://dictionary.cambridge.org/us/dictionary/english/model (accessed February 2, 2016).

The Council of the European Union. 2002. Council resolution of 27 June 2002 on lifelong learning. *Official Journal of the European Communities* C 163/161-C 163/163.

Frenk, J., L. Chen, Z. A. Bhutta, J. Cohen, N. Crisp, T. Evans, H. Fineberg, P. Garcia, Y. Ke, P. Kelley, B. Kistnasamy, A. Meleis, D. Naylor, A. Pablos-Mendez, S. Reddy, S. Scrimshaw, J. Sepulveda, D. Serwadda, and H. Zurayk. 2010. Health professionals for a new century: Transforming education to strengthen health systems in an interdependent world. *Lancet* 376(9756):1923-1958.

HHS (U.S. Department of Health and Human Services). 2016. *Healthypeople.gov: Disparities.* http://www.healthypeople.gov/2020/about/foundation-health-measures/Disparities (accessed January 28, 2016).

Kolb, D. A. 1984. *Experiential learning: Experience as the source of learning and development.* Englewood Cliffs, NJ: Prentice-Hall.

TUFH (Towards Unity for Health). 2000. *Towards Unity for Health: Coordinating changes in health services and health professions practice and education.* Geneva, Switzerland: WHO.

WHO (World Health Organization). 1987. *Community-based education of health personnel. Report of a WHO study group.* WHO technical report series 746. Geneva, Switzerland: WHO.

WHO. 1998. *Health promotion glossary.* Geneva, Switzerland: WHO.

WHO. 2002. *Community participation in local health and sustainability development: Approaches and techniques.* Copenhagen, Denmark: WHO.

WHO. 2008a. *Interprofessional education and collaborative practice glossary.* http://caipe.org.uk/silo/files/who-interprofessional-education-and-collaborative-practice-iecpglossary.doc (accessed September 22, 2016).

WHO. 2008b. *The world health report 2008. Primary health care: Now more than ever.* Geneva, Switzerland: WHO.

WHO. 2010. *Framework for action on interprofessional education and collaborative practice.* Geneva, Switzerland: WHO.

WHO. 2011. *Health systems strengthening glossary.* http://www.who.int/healthsystems/hss_glossary/en (accessed September 22, 2016.

WHO. 2016a. *Health systems: Equity.* http://www.who.int/healthsystems/topics/equity/en (accessed February 2, 2016).

WHO. 2016b. *Social determinants of health.* http://www.who.int/topics/social_determinants/en (accessed February 2, 2016).

Acknowledgments

The committee recognizes the efforts of several individuals whose contributions fostered discussion, enhanced the report's quality, and provided expert advice and opinions to inform the committee. With gratitude for their willingness to speak at the Open Session meeting on September 15, 2015, the committee members would like to thank: David Brown, Joanna Cain, Brigit Carter, Elizabeth Doerr, Kira Fortune, Pedro J. Greer, Lillian Holloway, Onelia Lage, Pierre LaRamée, Angelo McClain, Susan Scrimshaw, Sara Willems, and Shanita Williams.

The committee offers great appreciation for the consultants to the committee: Susan Scrimshaw, co-chair of the Global Forum on Innovation in Health Professional Education, and Sara Willems, author of the paper presented in Appendix A of the report; Karen Anderson, National Academies of Sciences, Engineering, and Medicine staff consultant; and Rona Briere, consultant editor.

The committee members would like to acknowledge the hard work of the study staff. Special appreciation goes to Patricia Cuff, study director, for her tireless efforts, keen dedication to the study, and adept skills. The committee also thanks Megan Perez, research associate; Bridget Callaghan, research assistant; and Patrick Kelley, board director of the Board on Global Health. In addition, the committee is grateful to the Academies Research Center, in particular Daniel Bearss and Rebecca Morgan, for conducting the literature review that provided the basis for Appendix A of the report.

Finally, the committee acknowledges its appreciation to the sponsors of this study; without their financial support, this study would not have been possible.

Summary

The World Health Organization (WHO) defines social determinants of health as "the conditions in which people are born, grow, work, live, and age, and the wider set of forces and systems shaping the conditions of daily life" (WHO, 2016a). These forces and systems include economic policies, development agendas, cultural and social norms, social policies, and political systems. Health inequities, "the unfair and avoidable differences in health between groups of people within countries and between countries" (WHO, 2016b), stem from the social determinants of health and result in stark differences in health and health outcomes. Other terms used to describe such differences reflect the countries in which they are used. In the United States, for example, the term "disparities" is often interpreted as racial or ethnic disparities (HHS, 2016) involving structural racism and other forms of unfair and unjust discrimination that create gaps in health among segments of the population. In the United Kingdom, the term "inequalities" is used to describe differences in health among groups based on socioeconomic conditions (Marmot and Allen, 2014). A consistent message embedded in each definition, regardless of its usage, is that if the underlying causes of disease and ill health are not addressed, the risk of perpetuating a cycle of inequity, disparity, and inequality will remain for generations to come.

PURPOSE OF THIS STUDY

Educating health professionals about the social determinants of health generates awareness of the potential root causes of ill health and the importance of addressing them in and with communities. The individual sponsors[1] of the Global Forum on Innovation in Health Professional Education of the Institute of Medicine (IOM) of the National Academies of Sciences, Engineering, and Medicine that called for a study of this topic expect greater awareness to lead to more effective strategies for improving health and health care for underserved populations now and in the future. Based on this premise, a diverse committee of experts was tasked with developing a high-level framework for educating health professionals to address the social determinants of health. Such a framework would draw on lessons learned by educators working in this sphere. It would also include elements of relevant frameworks and ideas advanced by international thought leaders with respect to their vision for health professional education. Additionally, the framework would consider health professional education in the social determinants of health across the learning continuum, from foundational education through continuing professional development.

DEFINING HEALTH PROFESSIONALS

Health professionals are classified and defined in the International Labour Organization's International Standard Classification of Occupations, which is accepted and used by WHO as the reference for its policy resolutions and technical guidelines. While this list does not capture the full breadth of professions making up the health workforce, it does illustrate the point that health professionals are not a homogeneous group. Rather, they differ in the nature and scope of their roles, responsibilities, and functions in promoting, preventing, curing, rehabilitating, and palliating within a holistic health system. This system also employs health professionals as educators, administrators, public health advocates, researchers, and policy makers. Embedded within a holistic health system are caregivers and others, such as community health workers, who do not fit the classic definition of a health professional.[2] In addition, a large segment of the health workforce is immersed in clinical practice environments. These clinical workers have an orientation to health systems that emphasizes disease-based, curative models of care for treating individual patients. Their role in addressing the social determinants of health is complementary to that of population health specialists, who focus on health promotion and disease prevention within communities and populations. In essence, everyone involved in the health arena has a role in addressing the social determinants of health.

---

[1] For the full list of sponsors of the Global Forum on Innovation in Health Professional Education and also of this study, please see Appendix C. The sponsors represent 18 different professions and 9 countries.

[2] Based on the statement of task for this study, the focus of this committee was on educating health professionals.

CREATING LIFELONG LEARNERS

Making the social determinants of health a core component of all health professionals' lifelong learning pathways will engender in them the competence, skill, and passion to take action, independent of their role and position in the health system, on these crucial contributors to individual and community health, and enhance their ability to identify, engage, and partner with others to take this action. The social determinants of health can and should be integral to all health professional education and training. As they progress though their educational programs and their careers, health professionals can gain greater understanding of the social determinants of health and how to partner within and outside of the health sector and with communities through formal and informal continuing professional development.

While creating lifelong learners is frequently seen as starting with admission into a health professional program, in reality the process starts long before that and continues well beyond retirement (CEU, 2002; Perels et al., 2009). University–community partnerships that create quality primary and secondary education programs in vulnerable communities provide exposure of community organizations to health professional students while also potentially embedding a desire to learn in young minds. Additionally, investment in early childhood development and education will increase the pool of potential candidates for health workforce education and training, which could be further enhanced through bridging programs designed to help adults enter the health workforce later in life. With greater professional maturity and a deepening understanding of the economic, political, and social causes of health disparities, health professionals gain further appreciation of and skills for addressing the social determinants of health, both individually and collectively.

THE ROLE OF EDUCATORS

University faculty members who are motivated to offer experiential, cross-sectoral, and interprofessional educational opportunities often confront significant barriers to acquiring the training necessary to provide these opportunities. Faculty development is a key requirement for obtaining relevant educational competencies and skills, which must also be matched by career pathways and rewards from academic leadership. While many health professional schools embrace experiential, cross-sectoral, and interprofessional education in partnership with communities, many have limited ability and desire to adopt incentives that would encourage faculty to become trained in this area (Calleson et al., 2002; Frenk et al., 2010; Goldstein and Bearman, 2011; Meleis, 2016).

Educators in clinical settings also have a role to play in addressing the social determinants of health as they reinforce concepts learned by students and trainees during community and didactic educational experiences. In this way, students transitioning into practice see the impacts of the social determinants of health on the health and well-being of individual patients. All educators thus need to have a common understanding of how social, economic, and policy decisions affect populations and can negatively impact individual health outcomes.

Engaging educators (clinical and nonclinical) from different communities offers numerous benefits. Expanded diversity enhances creativity and performance gains while providing a wider array of culturally and linguistically distinct role models. Having educators from diverse backgrounds also increases the likelihood that a student will identify a mentor with personal and cultural characteristics similar to his or her own.

THE IMPORTANCE OF PARTNERSHIPS

Partnerships are key to effectively addressing the social determinants of health. These partnerships entail close working relationships among policy makers, educators, representatives of the health and nonhealth professions, community organizations, and community members. They also involve strong linkages between nonclinical faculty and clinical faculty or preceptors so that experiences in and with communities related to the social determinants of health are reinforced during clinical rotations. Through such partnerships, health professionals gain exposure to the broader social, political, and environmental context that influences the health and health outcomes of individuals, populations, and communities. Innovative forms of education consolidate the unique aspects and experiences of each partner. Learners are challenged to solve problems and make new connections through exposure to other professions, sectors, and populations. Bidirectional linkages between partners reinforce equality in the partnership, which can be strengthened through organizational support.

A UNIFYING FRAMEWORK

The committee's review of the salient literature supports the need for a holistic, consistent, and coherent framework that can align the education, health, and other sectors, in partnership with communities, to educate health professionals in the social determinants of health. The outcome of such an education framework would differ based on the learner's position within the education continuum, from foundational (where the emphasis would be on broad exposure of students to and understanding of the social determinants of health) to continuing professional development (where health professionals would continue to learn from and with others to take action on the social determinants of health). Once trained, these individuals would become enlightened change agents competent to serve as faculty for students and peers to expand education on the social determinants of health. Ideally, they would be drawn from diverse communities.

One high-level assessment of health professional education posits that enlightened change agents are produced through transformative learning (Frenk et al., 2010). Instead of passive intake of facts, such learning emphasizes active participation in educational activities that build creative thinking and decision making, as well as competencies in collaboration. This notion heavily influenced the committee's development of the framework presented in this report, informed as well by ideas formulated by the WHO Commission on Social Determinants of Health. The Commission, comprising international thought leaders, policy makers, and representatives of civil society, produced a report emphasizing that poor health of certain individuals and groups is due to inequities caused by unequal distribution of power, income, goods, and services (WHO, 2008a). The Commission produced a conceptual framework for action on the social determinants of health that captures these ideas (Solar and Irwin, 2010). Heads of government, ministers, and government representatives from 120 member states used the Commission's framework and its other publications to draft their Rio Political Declaration on Social Determinants of Health (WHO, 2011a). In the Rio Declaration, the signatories affirm their "determination to achieve social and health equity through action on social determinants of health and well-being by a comprehensive intersectoral approach" (Marmot et al., 2013; WHO, 2011a, p. 1). They also emphasize that "health equity is a shared responsibility and requires the engagement of all sectors of government, of all segments of society, and of all members of the international community, in an 'all for equity' and 'health for all' global action" (WHO, 2011a, p. 1).

These global documents, along with ten relevant frameworks, programmatic examples of education in the social determinants of health described in the literature, presentations at a public meeting held by the committee, and the expert knowledge of the committee members formed the basis for the framework described below.

THE FRAMEWORK

The primary goal of creating partnerships and lifelong learners who desire more in-depth understanding of the social determinants of health is reflected in the committee's framework, presented in Figure S-1. This framework captures education at all levels, from foundational to gradu-

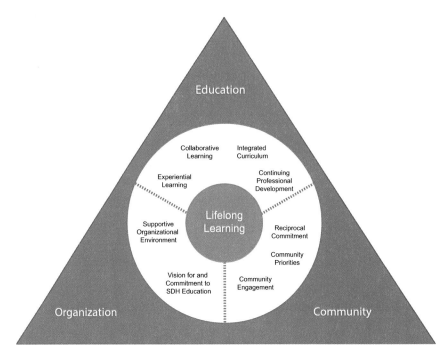

FIGURE S-1 Framework for lifelong learning for health professionals in understanding and addressing the social determinants of health.
NOTE: SDH = social determinants of health.

ate to continuing professional development. This education, which applies transformative learning techniques, is built around three domains:

1. education
2. community
3. organization

In Figure S-1, these three domains reside within a triangle signifying constant interaction among them. The white circle within the triangle contains nine domain components separated by dotted lines indicating that while these components apply predominantly to a particular domain, they can be applied to any of the domains. Lifelong learning is situated in the center of the framework, emphasizing its importance in the educational pathway of health professionals toward understanding and addressing the social determinants of health. Each of the three domains and its primary components are discussed in the sections below.

Education

The education domain is located at the top of the triangle in Figure S-1 to indicate that the framework is primarily about education. Listed within this domain are four components that education in the social determinants of health should include (see Box S-1). Education should be experiential, integrated, and collaborative across the learning continuum, including continuing professional development. A desired outcome for health professional students in the early stages of professional education would be to demonstrate an understanding of how social, political, and economic factors determine the health and health outcomes of individuals, communities, and populations. For clinical faculty, the outcome would be to demonstrate an understanding of how the social determinants of health are incorporated into clinical care. And for nonclinical faculty, the outcome would be improved pedagogy for educating students in the social determinants of health; their impacts on individual, community, and population health; and the role of key partners in improving the conditions that lead to inequities. Clinical and nonclinical faculty who work together can reinforce important messages about the social determinants of health while validating the importance of partnering to take action.

BOX S-1
Components of the Education Domain

Experiential learning
- Applied learning
- Community engagement
- Performance assessment

Collaborative learning
- Problem/project-based learning
- Student engagement
- Critical thinking

Integrated curriculum
- Interprofessional
- Cross-sectoral
- Longitudinally organized

Continuing professional development
- Faculty development
- Interprofessional workplace learning

In concurrence with member states' call for action on the social determinants of health (as expressed in the Rio Declaration), numerous provider organizations and educational associations, as well as individual faculty members, programs, and universities, are moving forward with activities to demonstrate action on the social determinants of health. While these efforts may add value, the risk of eroding the trust of vulnerable communities is very real. Thus, it is essential to understand a community's issues before acting on the social determinants of health through well-thought-out partnerships. Achieving consistency through a unified framework can help ensure that all health professionals understand the underlying social, economic, and political causes of poor mental and physical health among individuals and populations and are able to address these issues in a coordinated manner. Accordingly, the committee makes the following recommendation:

Recommendation 1: Health professional educators should use the framework presented in this report as a guide for creating lifelong learners who appreciate the value of relationships and collaborations for understanding and addressing community-identified needs and for strengthening community assets.

To demonstrate effective implementation of the framework, health professional educators should

- publish literature on analyses of and lessons learned from curricula that offer learning opportunities that are responsive to the evolving needs and assets of local communities; and
- document case studies of health professional advocacy using a health-in-all-policies approach.[3]

Community

Partnerships with communities are an essential part of educating health professionals in the social determinants of health. Three domain components would move education in this direction (see Box S-2). A reciprocal commitment ensures that the community is an equal partner in any initiative undertaken. The commitment is heavily based on community-identified priorities and real community engagement that are the second and third components of this domain. It is through shifts in power from health

---

[3] "Health in all policies" denotes a policy or reform designed to achieve healthier communities by integrating public health actions with primary care and by pursuing healthy public policies across sectors (WHO, 2008b, 2011b).

BOX S-2
Components of the Community Domain

Reciprocal commitment
- Community assets
- Willingness to engage
- Networks
- Resources

Community priorities
- Evaluation of health impacts toward equity and well-being

Community engagement
- Workforce diversity
- Recruitment, retention

---

professionals to community members and organizations that communities share in the responsibility for developing strategies for the creation of learning opportunities that can advance health equity based on community priorities and build upon community assets.

As suggested earlier, building pipelines to higher education in the health professions in underserved communities is a tested means of expanding the pool of viable candidates who have themselves been negatively affected by the social determinants of health. And while applications and admissions of such candidates may increase, equal emphasis on retaining them once they have been accepted into a program is essential, as is recruiting and retaining faculty from similarly underserved communities.

> **Recommendation 2: To prepare health professionals to take action on the social determinants of health in, with, and across communities, health professional and educational associations and organizations at the global, regional, and national levels should apply the concepts embodied in the framework in partnering with communities to increase the inclusivity and diversity of the health professional student body and faculty.**

To enable action on this recommendation, health professional education and training institutions should support pipelines to higher education in the health professions in underserved communities, thus expanding the pool of viable candidates who have themselves been negatively affected by the social determinants of health.

Organization

The two components of this domain (shown in Box S-3) emphasize a commitment to addressing the social determinants of health and creating an environment that will support the sort of understanding and actions discussed under the education domain. How committed an organization is to addressing the social determinants of health is reflected in its founding and guiding policies, strategies, education programs, and leadership-promoted activities. And while the actual words "social determinants of health" may not always appear in its documents, other relevant terms, such as "social justice," "disparities," "equity," "diversity," and "inclusivity," can reflect an organization's commitment to education in the social determinants of health for students and employees.

> **Recommendation 3: Governments and individual ministries (e.g., signatories of the Rio Declaration), health professional and educational associations and organizations, and community groups should foster an enabling environment that supports and values the integration of the framework's principles into their mission, culture, and work.**

To implement this recommendation, national governments, individual ministries, and health professional and educational associations and organizations should review, map, and align their educational and professional vision, mission, and standards to include the social determinants of health as described in the framework. The following actions would demonstrate organizational support for enhancing competency for addressing the social determinants of health:

BOX S-3
Components of the Organization Domain

Vision for and commitment to education in the social determinants of health
- Policies, strategies, and program reviews
- Resources
- Infrastructure
- Promotion/career pathways

Supportive organizational environment
- Transformative learning
- Dissemination of pedagogical research
- Faculty development/continuing professional development

- Produce and effectively disseminate case studies and evaluations on the use of the framework, integrating lessons learned to build and strengthen work on health professional education in the social determinants of health.
- Work with relevant government bodies to support and promote health professional education in the social determinants of health by aligning policies, planning, and financing and investments.
- Introduce accreditation of health professional education where it does not exist and strengthen it where it does.
- Design and implement continuing professional development programs for faculty and teaching staff that promote health equity and are relevant to the evolving health and health care needs and priorities of local communities.
- Support experiential learning opportunities that are interprofessional and cross-sectoral and involve partnering with communities.

FITTING THE FRAMEWORK INTO A CONCEPTUAL MODEL

Applying concepts and ideas from multiple sources, the committee developed a conceptual model (see Figure S-2) for visualizing how the framework fits within a broader societal context (Frenk et al., 2010; HHS, 2010; Solar and Irwin, 2010; Sousa et al., 2013; WHO, 2006, 2008a, 2011a). The model depicts how social, political, and economic factors (i.e., the structures in which populations live) influence intermediary determinants (i.e., material and psychosocial circumstances, behavioral and/or biological factors, and the health system itself) that ultimately determine health equity and the well-being of populations. Communities and the future health workforce are influenced by the structural and intermediary determinants that form the environment for educating health professionals in the social determinants of health.

Positioned in the center of the model is the committee's framework. To the left of the framework is the *population/future health workforce*,[4] which forms the pipeline for the education and production of future health professionals. Through a transformative learning approach, health professionals, students, and trainees gain an understanding of how to establish equal partnerships with communities, other sectors, and other professions for action on the social determinants of health. Those who are educated

---

[4] The population/future health workforce includes the pool of eligible students. The development of this workforce starts with primary and secondary education to encourage a new generation of health workers at the pre-entry stage. It also includes adults who might enter the health workforce from other sectors, as well as current health workers looking to expand their knowledge or change their employment position.

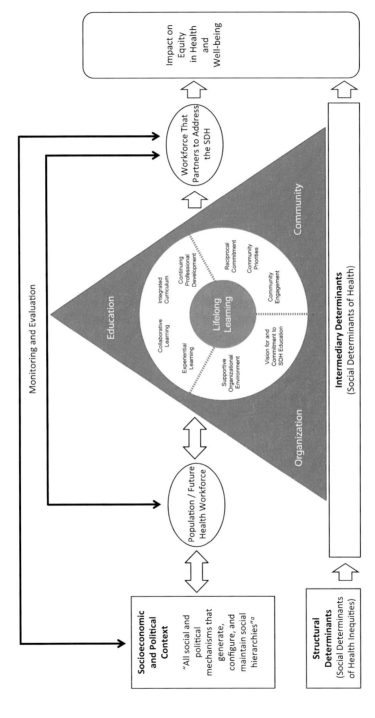

FIGURE S-2 Conceptual model for strengthening health professional education in the social determinants of health.

NOTE: SDH = social determinants of health.

a Solar and Irwin, 2010, p. 5.

in line with the framework also gain competency in addressing health system complexities within an increasingly global and interconnected world, thereby becoming part of a *workforce that partners to address the social determinants of health* toward the ultimate goal of achieving *impact on equity in health and well-being.*

Measuring the degree to which health professionals understand and partner to address the social determinants of health before and after undergoing transformative education in the social determinants of health is a way of determining the proximal impact of the framework. However, the desired impact of the framework is on the more distal outcomes of improving the health and well-being of individuals, communities, and populations. Using established methodology for analyzing cause-and-effect relationships between educational interventions and these distal outcomes will be critical to building an evidence base on the effects of the framework on both learning and health outcomes.

BUILDING THE EVIDENCE BASE

While numerous articles describe student activities within communities to address the social determinants of health, few publications offer evidence beyond student outcomes for analyzing the value to communities of such health professional education. The gap is due in part to a lack of well-established methods for conducting such an analysis. Reports outlining lessons learned from educational experiences designed to impact the social determinants of health are useful for understanding potential barriers to partnerships, but do not provide guidance for researchers or evaluators seeking to impact community outcomes. Further evidence that goes beyond self-examination is needed to inform the education of health professionals. Obtaining objective and subjective input from community partners would help build the evidence base for learning in and with communities while impacting the social determinants of health and inform best practices for lifelong learning.

> **Recommendation 4: Governments, health professional and educational associations and organizations, and community organizations should use the committee's framework and model to guide and support evaluation research aimed at identifying and illustrating effective approaches for learning about the social determinants of health in and with communities while improving health outcomes, thereby building the evidence base.**

To demonstrate full and equal partnerships, health professional and educational associations and organizations and community partners should prepare their respective networks to engage with one another in a systematic, comprehensive inquiry aimed at building the evidence base.

MOVING FORWARD

Achieving lasting impacts on the social determinants of health will require action at multiple levels from multiple stakeholders. This report addresses one narrowly defined area—health professional education—while stressing the importance of strategic partnerships that extend beyond the walls of health professional schools. Extensive detail on the partners is beyond the scope of this report but warrants mentioning to encourage future studies, possibly with a broader mandate, focused in greater depth on these other critical stakeholders. One such key group is community health workers. These individuals usually come from the community served, are culturally and linguistically competent, and enjoy a high level of trust in the community. They are increasingly serving as members of health care teams and as facilitators of community engagement and training of health science students in community perspectives (Torres et al., 2014). Other critical groups include health workers educated and trained at community colleges and vocational training institutes, as well as representatives of nonhealth sectors such as education, labor, housing, transportation, urban planning, community development, and public policy.

Another crucial area for more thorough investigation is investment in health professional education. The committee recognizes that without adequate financial support and sustainable investment, the education envisioned in this report will remain predominantly a series of one-off, ad hoc efforts by motivated but often overburdened, undersupported individuals. And while a recommendation on funding is beyond the mandate and expertise of this committee, the following points are offered as considerations for future explorations of this topic.

First is the recognition that governments and ministries have the power to direct health professional education, and power brokers who control major resources within academic health centers and hospitals also have an important role in addressing the social determinants of health. By reallocating graduate education funding and examining the rules governing special tax status, for example, national governments can shift the focus of education and practice more toward community engagement. Similarly, ministries can direct the use of funds through educational requirements. Often such shifts require evidence demonstrating a return on investment relevant to a particular health system. For some this evidence will be financial savings, and for others it may involve tracking such indicators as the health and well-being of community residents and the social accountability of health professional schools (Annis et al., 2004; Boelen et al., 2012; Danaher, 2011; Ryan-Nicholls, 2004).

A second point is that funders of and payers for health professional education and research need to be part of any discussion moving forward. This group includes students, employers, governments, and foundations with a stake in how health professionals are educated to address the social determinants of health. Foundations exert influence through the activities they support. If these activities build the evidence base for interventions that educate students while benefiting communities socially and financially, those data empower students, communities, and educators to advocate for a redirection of funding. In the context of this report, such redirection could focus funds toward expanding opportunities that promote incorporation of the social determinants of health into community programs that also train current and future generations of health professionals.

A third point is that many stakeholder groups will need to advocate for greater educational focus on the social determinants of health based on the potential financial, social, and health benefits to society, although these groups should be prepared for resistance. One way to overcome this resistance would be to build a business case. To this end, more data are needed to demonstrate efficient and equitable outcomes attributable to health professionals being educated in the social determinants of health because such information is currently sparse.

Resistance to change is just one likely challenge faced by advocates. Another is ensuring appropriate engagement of communities, especially marginalized communities with low-income populations who have previously been used by academic institutions for research that has not benefited them or their communities. At times, students and health professionals with extremely limited experience and exposure to community engagement and the social determinants of health may push for interventions in a way that is counterproductive to building community relations. And while requirements under accreditation standards may force programs to offer interprofessional, cross-sector, community-engaged learning, proper leadership support and adequate training also are necessary, or the quality of the programs offered may fulfill the requirements but fail to inspire a desire for lifelong learning in how to mitigate the root causes of ill health and disease.

In closing, it is the committee's hope that leaders within health professional education who claim to already address elements of the framework will review their efforts in conjunction with staff, employees, students, and educators. These leaders could measure their success by evaluating the extent to which their educational interventions impact a desire for lifelong learning to better understand and act upon the social determinants of health in equal partnership with others.

REFERENCES

Annis, R., F. Racher, and M. Beattie. 2004. *Rural community health and well-being: A guide to action*. Brandon, Manitoba: Rural Development Institute. https://www.brandonu.ca/rdi/publication/rural-community-health-and-well-being-a-guide-to-action (accessed September 22, 2016).

Boelen, C., S. Dharamsi, and T. Gibbs. 2012. The social accountability of medical schools and its indicators. *Education for Health (Abingdon, England)* 25(3):180-194.

Calleson, D. C., S. D. Seifer, and C. Maurana. 2002. Forces affecting community involvement of AHCS: Perspectives of institutional and faculty leaders. *Academic Medicine* 77(1):72-81.

CEU (The Council of the European Union). 2002. Council resolution of 27 June 2002 on lifelong learning. *Official Journal of the European Union*. Brussels: C 163/1.

Danaher, A. 2011. *Reducing disparities and improving population health: The role of a vibrant community sector*. Toronto, ON: Wellesley Institute.

Frenk, J., L. Chen, Z. A. Bhutta, J. Cohen, N. Crisp, T. Evans, H. Fineberg, P. Garcia, Y. Ke, P. Kelley, B. Kistnasamy, A. Meleis, D. Naylor, A. Pablos-Mendez, S. Reddy, S. Scrimshaw, J. Sepulveda, D. Serwadda, and H. Zurayk. 2010. Health professionals for a new century: Transforming education to strengthen health systems in an interdependent world. *Lancet* 376(9756):1923-1958.

Goldstein, A. O., and R. S. Bearman. 2011. Community engagement in US and Canadian medical schools. *Advances in Medical Education and Practice* 2:43-49.

HHS (U.S. Department of Health and Human Services). 2010. *Healthy People 2020*. Washington, DC: HHS. http://www.healthypeople.gov/sites/default/files/HP2020_brochure_with_LHI_508_FNL.pdf (accessed January 11, 2016).

HHS. 2016. *Healthypeople.gov: Disparities*. http://www.healthypeople.gov/2020/about/foundation-health-measures/Disparities (accessed January 28, 2016).

Marmot, M., and J. J. Allen. 2014. Social determinants of health equity. *American Journal of Public Health* 104(Suppl. 4):S517-S519.

Marmot, M., A. Pellegrini Filho, J. Vega, O. Solar, and K. Fortune. 2013. Action on social determinants of health in the Americas. *Revista Panamericana de Salud Pública* 34(6):379-384.

Meleis, A. I. 2016. Interprofessional education: A summary of reports and barriers to recommendations. *Journal of Nursing Scholarship* 48(1):106-112.

Perels, F., M. Merget-Kullmann, M. Wende, B. Schmitz, and C. Buchbinder. 2009. Improving self-regulated learning of preschool children: Evaluation of training for kindergarten teachers. *British Journal of Educational Psychology* 79(Pt 2):311-327.

Ryan-Nicholls, K. 2004. Rural Canadian community health and quality of life: Testing a workbook to determine priorities and move to action. *Rural Remote Health* 4(2):278.

Solar, O., and A. Irwin. 2010. *A conceptual framework for action on the social determinants of health. Social determinants of health discussion paper 2 (policy and practice)*. Geneva, Switzerland: WHO. http://www.who.int/sdhconference/resources/Conceptualframeworkforactionon SDH_eng.pdf (accessed September 22, 2016).

Sousa, A., R. M. Scheffler, J. Nyoni, and T. Boerma. 2013. A comprehensive health labour market framework for universal health coverage. *Bulletin of the World Health Organization* 91(11):892-894. http://www.who.int/bulletin/volumes/91/11/13-118927.pdf (accessed September 22, 2016).

Torres, S., R. Labonté, D. L. Spitzer, C. Andrew, and C. Amaratunga. 2014. Improving health equity: The promising role of community health workers in Canada. *Healthcare Policy* 10(1):73-85.

WHO (World Health Organization). 2006. *The world health report 2006: Working together for health.* Geneva, Switzerland: WHO. http://www.who.int/whr/2006/en (accessed September 22, 2016).

WHO. 2008a. *Closing the gap in a generation: Health equity through action on the social determinants of health, final report.* Geneva, Switzerland: WHO Commission on Social Determinants of Health.

WHO. 2008b. *The world health report 2008. Primary health care: Now more than ever.* Geneva, Switzerland: WHO.

WHO. 2011a. *Rio political declaration on social determinants of health.* Adopted at the World Conference on the Social Determinants of Health, Rio de Janeiro, Brazil. Geneva, Switzerland: WHO. http://www.who.int/sdhconference/declaration/Rio_political_declaration.pdf?ua=1 (accessed September 22, 2016).

WHO. 2011b. *Health systems strengthening glossary.* http://www.who.int/healthsystems/hss_glossary/en (accessed September 22, 2016).

WHO. 2016a. *Social determinants of health.* http://www.who.int/social_determinants/en (accessed February 2, 2016).

WHO. 2016b. *Social determinants of health.* http://www.who.int/topics/social_determinants/en (accessed February 2, 2016).

1

Introduction

SUMMARY

This chapter sets the stage for the rest of the report, which presents a holistic, comprehensive framework in response to the study committee's statement of task. Critical to this framework is an understanding of the term "social determinants of health," which all health professionals have a role in addressing. Some health professionals will specialize in the care of individuals, while others will focus on population-based interventions designed to impact the health of communities. Regardless of this orientation, all health professionals need to develop an understanding during their foundational education and training of the outside forces that impact a person's, community's, or population's health and well-being. Subsequent chapters offer concrete examples of programs and frameworks addressing elements of the social determinants of health, while this chapter focuses on theoretical constructs put forth by researchers and high-level commissions that form much of the basis for the committee's framework.

In an era of pronounced human migration, changing demographics, and growing financial gaps between rich and poor, foundational education programs for health professionals need to equip their graduates with at least a fundamental understanding of how the conditions and circumstances in which individuals and populations exist affect mental and physical health. Professionals who specialize in health care, often as providers, will likely have an individual-, disease-, and treatment-focused orientation to health systems, while those who specialize in public health will focus predominantly on prevention and wellness efforts aimed at communities and populations. Yet regardless of their role, responsibilities, and health system orientation, all health professionals are part of a holistic system in an interconnected world in which they increasingly must rely on others within and outside of the health professions. Thus, they must have an understanding of outside forces that influence decisions affecting patients and populations. Such outside forces include predetermined circumstances based on an individual's or community's access to money, power, and resources, as well as local, national, and global policies. Health professional students who are exposed to these concepts in ways that inspire further learning are better positioned to educate future generations of health professionals, having experienced this education firsthand. However, even the most experienced educator cannot alone provide students with all facets of education necessary for a complete understanding of what the World Health Organization (WHO) terms the "social determinants of health" as "the conditions in which people are born, grow, live, work, and age, including the health system" (2016a).

Educators need to partner with others to provide this sort of education. By partnering with other professionals, professions, sectors, and communities, educators can model the sorts of activities that health professionals wish to pursue in their respective roles as providers or population health specialists, or in other selected career paths. Because the time health professionals spend in foundational education and training is small compared with career-based education, it is also the job of educators to instill a desire in their students for greater learning about the social determinants of health. With continued formal and informal learning, health professionals are best positioned to work with others in taking action on the social determinants of health to improve the health and well-being of individuals, communities, and populations.

It is in this context that the individual sponsors of the Global Forum on Innovation in Health Professional Education of the Institute of Medicine (IOM) of the National Academies of Sciences, Engineering, and Medicine (see Appendix C) requested that the IOM convene a committee to develop a high-level framework for educating health professionals to address the social determinants of health.

STUDY CHARGE

The study committee comprised 10 experts from diverse backgrounds, professions, and expertise who convened for 4 days to review the literature and hear public testimony on how health professionals are currently being educated to address the social determinants of health, and to develop a framework for better educating health professionals in this critical arena. As defined in its statement of task (see Box 1-1), the committee was to focus on experiential learning opportunities in and with communities in developing this framework. The framework would draw on a variety of outlined perspectives spanning the continuum of health professional learning, from foundational to graduate education to continuing professional development. The global and diverse makeup of the individual sponsors and members of the Global Forum is reflected in the committee's composition. As requested by the sponsors, the framework would be general in nature to suit multiple contexts around the world but adaptable for local applications that might differ by setting and circumstances.

STUDY APPROACH

The committee's approach to carrying out its statement of task encompassed

- a balanced committee of experts vetted for biases and conflicts of interest;
- a commissioned paper examining existing programs and curricula designed to educate health professionals to address the social determinants of health (see Appendix A);

BOX 1-1
Statement of Task

An ad hoc committee under the auspices of the Institute of Medicine will conduct a study to explore how the education of health professionals is currently addressing the social determinants of health in and with communities. Based on these findings, the committee will develop a framework for how the education of health professionals for better understanding the social determinants of health could be strengthened across the learning continuum.

The committee can consider a variety of perspectives—that could include partnerships, finances and sustainability, experiential learning, continuing professional development, faculty development, policies, systems, and/or health literacy—in preparation of a brief report containing recommendations on how to strengthen health professional education in and with vulnerable communities by addressing the social determinants of health.

- 1 day of open testimony from outside experts, which supplemented the knowledge of the committee members (see Appendix B for the agenda for this session and Appendix D for speaker biographies);
- 3 days of closed-door deliberations during which the committee agreed on a framework, a conceptual model, and recommendations; and
- virtual meetings during which the recommendations presented in this report were finalized.

UNDERSTANDING THE SOCIAL DETERMINANTS OF HEALTH

The conditions encompassed by WHO's definition of the social determinants of health are typically predetermined based on an individual's or community's access to money, power, and resources—which are also influenced by policy choices—from local to global contexts. They are most responsible for the "unfair and avoidable differences in health status seen within and between countries" (WHO, 2016a). A girl born in Sierra Leone who survives to the age of 5 is halfway through her predicted life span by the time she reaches age 17, whereas a girl born on the same day in Japan can expect to live into her 80s and will likely not die before she turns 5. This is the case because, unlike her counterpart in Sierra Leone who faces an under-5 mortality rate of 316 per 1,000 live births, the girl in Japan has only a 5 in 1,000 probability of dying before she reaches her fifth birthday (Marmot, 2005). These are the sobering messages of Sir Michael Marmot, who describes the "gross inequalities in health" (p. 1) that exist among countries but are also evident within even the wealthiest of nations. Marmot and others have shed light on how compiled morbidity and mortality data at the national level can obscure intergroup disparities within a country (Braveman and Tarimo, 2002; *The Economist*, 2012; Marmot, 2005).

In the United Kingdom, population differences often are referred to as "inequalities" among groups based on socioeconomic conditions (Marmot and Allen, 2014). In the United States, for example, the term "disparities" is often interpreted as racial and ethnic differences in health care (HHS, 2016a). "Health equity" is a third term that, according to Wirth and colleagues (2006) in their guide to monitoring the Millennium Development Goals, is based on simple notions of fairness and distributive justice. The authors further delineate nuances between disparities and inequities, saying, "when disparities are strongly and systematically associated with certain social group characteristics such as level of wealth or education, whether one lives in a city or rural area, they are termed inequities" (Wirth et al., 2006). All of these contextual nuances of gross inequalities in health have similar origins in the social determinants of health.

A landmark study by McGinnis and Foege (1993) identifies and quantifies causes of death in the year 1990. What is revealing about their research is that half of the deaths could be attributed to nongenetic factors such as tobacco, diet/activity patterns, alcohol, and firearms. Since that time, others have categorized these factors into major domains that include (1) individual behaviors, (2) social environment or characteristics, (3) environmental conditions, and (4) health services and health care (CDC, 2014; HHS, 2016b; McGinnis et al., 2002). Link and Phelan (1995) draw connections between social conditions and risk factors similar to those identified by McGinnis and Foege—what these authors refer to as the "risks of the risks." They argue that to focus on individual treatment strategies would be to miss the opportunity for broad-based societal interventions.

Given the ways in which race and socioeconomic status combine to affect health and disease rates (Williams, 1999), many researchers and public health advocates now identify racism as a determinant of health (Jones et al., 2009; Markwick et al., 2014; Reading and Wien, 2009). A meta-analysis of the literature examining the impacts of racism on mental and physical health outcomes uncovered 293 studies published between 1983 and 2013 (Paradies et al., 2015). The analysis revealed that racism is associated with poorer mental and physical health after controlling for age, sex, birthplace, and education. While the vast majority of the articles in this review focus on the United States, WHO also is aware of the interactions among ethnicity, race, and health (WHO, 2014). A study cited in its *Review of Social Determinants and the Health Divide in the WHO European Region* shows that Roma children in the former Yugoslav Republic of Macedonia, Montenegro, and Serbia have the highest rates of stunting, which exceed 17 percent in each of those countries (Falkingham et al., 2012).

DIVERSITY AND INCLUSIVITY

There is growing awareness of the value of diversity in health professional education that goes beyond scholarships offered to underrepresented groups, and of the fact that such diversity could directly (e.g., through university–community partnerships) and indirectly (e.g., through faculty hiring and retention policies) impact the social determinants of health. Approaches for increasing diversity and enhancing the mix of backgrounds that make up the health and education workforce vary (Dogra et al., 2009; Price et al., 2009). Dogra and colleagues (2009) offer suggestions for developing cultural diversity in education by integrating institutional policies, curriculum content, faculty development, and assessment. While valuable, the need for culturally similar health professionals that reflect the changing demographics would add greater credibility to these efforts

(Cohen et al., 2002; Gijón-Sánchez et al., 2010; Grumbach and Mendoza, 2008; Phillips and Malone, 2014). In this regard, Price and colleagues (2009) suggest that attention to the structural barriers, such as retention efforts and mentorship, could improve the psychological climate and structural diversity of the institution. Structural changes can increase the number of students from diverse backgrounds; however, some argue that increasing diversity does not go far enough. They contend that increasing the diversity of educational organizations and schools does not necessarily create an environment of inclusivity where all students, faculty, staff, and others feel safe interacting and working within their respective environments (Elliot et al., 2013; Haney, 2015; Mulé et al., 2009). With greater attention to equity, the ideals for diversity found in mission statements, visions, and policies can more likely be realized for individuals particularly those from marginalized communities.

THE WORLD HEALTH ORGANIZATION'S COMMISSION ON SOCIAL DETERMINANTS OF HEALTH

The WHO Commission on Social Determinants of Health—comprising policy makers, researchers, and representatives of civil society from around the globe—analyzed the evidence for concluding that the poor health of certain individuals and groups is due to inequities caused by unequal distribution of power, income, goods, and services (WHO, 2008). Based on this analysis, the Commission's report calls on WHO and its member states to "lead global action on the social determinants of health with the aim of achieving health equity." Such unfairness, the report contends, dramatically impacts the ability of individuals and communities to access health-promoting resources such as health care, schools, education, safe working environments, and healthy living conditions (WHO, 2008). The report offers three overarching recommendations for moving the world toward achieving health equity within a generation:

1. Improve daily living conditions.
2. Tackle the inequitable distribution of power, money, and resources.
3. Measure and understand the problem and assess the impact of action.

The first of these recommendations specifically calls for policies to achieve goals that would improve the well-being of girls and women as reflected in the Millennium Development Goals. It also emphasizes the importance of early child development and education and the creation of conditions that would have positive impacts throughout an individual's life span. The second recommendation acknowledges the need to address

inequities, such as those between men and women, through good governance, adequate financing, and a strong public sector. The third recommendation is focused on establishment of a system of accountability both
within countries and globally.

LANCET COMMISSION ON
EDUCATION OF HEALTH PROFESSIONALS

Complementing the work of the WHO Commission, the *Lancet* convened global academic thought leaders to articulate a new vision for health
professional education (Frenk et al., 2010). The *Lancet* commissioners, too,
note glaring gaps and inequities in health both within and among countries.
They further express concern that health professionals are not graduating
with the sorts of competencies needed to understand how to combat such
disparities. To address this and other concerns, the commissioners recommend instructional and institutional strategies for reforming health professional education that, if adopted, would lead to transformative learning
and interdependence in education, respectively. The *Lancet* commissioners
posit that the purpose of transformative learning is to "produce enlightened change agents" (Frenk et al., 2010, p. 1924) and to create leaders.
Interdependence would involve the alignment of education and health systems; stronger and more stable networks, alliances, and partnerships; and
a broader perspective on learning that would encompass models, content,
and innovations from all countries and communities. These instructional
and institutional strategies would involve competency-based approaches
to instructional design that are global and collaborative and would place
particular emphasis on faculty development. The envisioned health workforce that would result from implementation of these strategies would be
better prepared to advocate with and for others, to partner with community
leaders to make positive change in their community, and to work toward
achieving equity in health and well-being for all populations.

MAKING THE CASE

Taking action on the social determinants of health as a core function
of health professionals' work holds promise for improving individual and
population health outcomes, leading in turn to significant financial benefits.
Congruent with these economic gains, however, Sir Michael Marmot stresses
that taking action to reduce health inequalities is a "matter of social justice"
(Allen et al., 2013; Marmot, 2005; Moscrop, 2012). Additionally, WHO
has made addressing the social determinants of health one of its six priority
areas (WHO, 2014), and recognizes that educating the health workforce to
promote health equity by addressing and taking action on the social deter-

minants of health is a fundamental requirement of the health and education systems (WHO, 2008, 2013a). Achieving this goal, however, is not just a matter of health workforce curriculum development. The 2006 WHO World Health report (WHO, 2006) and other influential reports highlight two connected and interdependent issues for health workforce education: (1) the critical shortages, maldistribution, and skill gaps of the current health workforce; and (2) the challenges entailed in educating and training the health workforce in many countries, including insufficient financial means, facilities, and numbers of educators to train an adequate, competent cadre of health workers (COGME, 1998; Ko et al., 2007; WHO, 2013b).

The adoption of the 2030 Agenda for Sustainable Development (UN, 2015) has provided the impetus and architecture for the movement of WHO (the United Nations agency responsible for health) and the United Nations Educational, Scientific and Cultural Organization (UNESCO, the United Nations agency responsible for education) into an era of closer collaboration. Emerging global and national strategies for developing human resources for health stress that education of the health workforce in the social determinants of health must be framed within a country's individual sociopolitical context and embedded in cross-sectoral efforts to promote heath equity (WHO, 2015a). The alignment of health, education, and development toward sustainable development goals has reinforced the need for such a cross-sectoral approach.

United Nations agencies recognize that standardized measurement and accountability will be required (MA4Health, 2015). The development of national health workforce accounts, including one for education, is integral to the WHO Global Strategy on Human Resources for Health (OECD et al., 2015; WHO, 2009, 2015b).

Many agencies and organizations, as well as individual educators, practitioners, and researchers, acknowledge that the complex nature of the social determinants of health is best addressed interprofessionally (Art et al., 2007; Bainbridge et al., 2014; Mihalynuk et al., 2007; Solar and Irwin, 2010). Such collaborations need to include not only an appropriate mix of health professionals and health sector workers, but also professionals and workers from other sectors (Allen et al., 2013; Art et al., 2007; Bainbridge et al., 2014; Lomazzi et al., 2016; Solar and Irwin, 2010). The effective application of interprofessional and cross-sectoral education has potential significant downstream consequences, not only in improving health outcomes, but also in reducing health inequalities and promoting health equity (Bollela et al., 2015). However, given the lack of racial and ethnic diversity in health professional education, a number of the health professions, and thus health professional teams, a key opportunity is missed to use workforce diversity as a way to eliminate health disparities (Cohen et al., 2002; Dapremont, 2012; Grumbach and Mendoza, 2008; HRSA, 2006; Price et al., 2005). The disparity between the diversity of teams and the diversity of the communities they serve undermines the effectiveness of the care and services provided.

ANSWERING THE CALL

On October 21, 2011, member states and stakeholders came together for the World Conference on the Social Determinants of Health. At that historic event, participants shared a global platform for dialogue on experiences related to policies and strategies aimed at reducing health inequities. It was here that the Rio Political Declaration on Social Determinants of Health[1] was adopted by the 120 member states, and discussion focused on how the recommendations of the WHO Commission on Social Determinants of Health (WHO, 2008), which laid the foundation for the Rio Political Declaration, could be taken forward. A goal of this effort was to create energy for country-driven efforts leading to national action plans and strategies (WHO, 2011).

Numerous governments and their ministries have responded to this call to action (Government of Canada, 2015; WHO, 2016b). In addition, a wide array of educational, health professional, and community associations and organizations from around the world have similarly called for action and have begun taking steps toward building a workforce competent to address the social determinants of health (Australian Medical Association, 2007; CMA, 2013; CORDIS, 2015; HHS, 2010c; IFMSA, 2014; Solar and Irwin, 2010; UNDP, 2013; WHO, 2014; WHPA, 2010). Foundations have been another powerful force in efforts addressing the social determinants of health (RWJF, 2008; WKKF, 2016).

A review of the literature (see Appendix A) reveals that educators are responding to the need to address the social determinants of health, but that many of these efforts are conducted uniprofessionally or with a small number of interacting professions, and the education is heavily weighted toward classroom activities. Additionally, experiential learning opportunities tend to be short-term, volunteer, and in the form of community service learning activities, and rural clinical settings are at times described as community-based education with no outreach into the community. While

---

[1] The Rio Political Declaration on Social Determinants of Health (WHO, 2011) is the formal statement of 120 heads of government, ministers, and government representatives that affirms their "determination to achieve social and health equity through action on social determinants of health and well-being by a comprehensive intersectoral approach" (Marmot et al., 2013; WHO, 2011, p. 1). It expresses their understanding that "health equity is a shared responsibility and requires the engagement of all sectors of government, of all segments of society, and of all members of the international community, in an 'all for equity' and 'health for all' global action" (p. 1).

each effort to address the social determinants of health is laudable and can add educational value if done well, a single isolated activity does not rise to the vision of the WHO or *Lancet* global health thought leaders. These commissions suggest a more comprehensive approach to educating health professionals that would draw on best practices of

- interprofessional education,
- community-engaged learning,
- experiential education, and
- health outcomes research.

Obstacles to incorporating any one of these approaches into health professional education have been fully explored. However, many health professional and educational organizations have found ways of facilitating each approach. These methods could be evaluated to determine the appropriateness of adapting them to health professional education addressing the social determinants of health, provided that faculty are appropriately trained and the community is prepared to partner.

REPORT STRUCTURE

In contrast to the theoretical discussion of the social determinants of health and health professional education presented in this chapter, Chapter 2 examines how educators and educational organizations and institutions are addressing the social determinants of health through different curricula and programs. The information in this chapter was informed by the background paper commissioned for this study (see Appendix A), whose authors reviewed the published literature specifically on education addressing the social determinants of health conducted in and with communities. Terms of reference for this paper, and accordingly the authors' literature search, were quite narrowly defined to reflect the scope of the committee's task.

Chapter 3 shifts from individual examples of education, networks, and partnerships to the broader concept of frameworks within which curricula and programs can be tailored to meet situational requirements. The committee reviewed numerous frameworks for this study. Chapter 3 describes ten of the most relevant structures, drawn from such areas as education, public health, community engagement, and social accountability. These structures capture various aspects of the committee's charge that informed its development of the framework and the recommendations supporting its implementation presented in this report. The committee's framework and recommendations, along with a conceptual model for strengthening health professional education in the social determinants of health, appear in the fourth and final chapter of this report.

REFERENCES

Allen, M., J. Allen, S. Hogarth, and M. Marmot. 2013. *Working for health equity: The role of health professionals.* London, UK: University College of London Institute of Health Policy.

Art, B., L. De Roo, and J. De Maeseneer. 2007. Towards Unity for Health utilising community-oriented primary care in education and practice. *Education for Health (Abingdon, England)* 20(2):74.

Australian Medical Association. 2007. *Social determinants of health and the prevention of health inequities—2007.* https://ama.com.au/position-statement/social-determinants-health-and-prevention-health-inequities-2007 (accessed February 1, 2016).

Bainbridge, L., S. Grossman, S. Dharamsi, J. Porter, and V. Wood. 2014. Engagement studios: Students and communities working to address the determinants of health. *Education for Health (Abingdon, England)* 27(1):78-82.

Bollela, V. R., A. C. Germani, H. de Holanda Campos, and E. M. Amaral. 2015. *Community-based education for the health professions: Learning from the Brazilian experience.* São Paulo, Brazil: Pan American Health Organization.

Braveman, P., and E. Tarimo. 2002. Social inequalities in health within countries: Not only an issue for affluent nations. *Social Science & Medicine* 54(11):1621-1635.

CDC (Centers for Disease Control and Prevention). 2014. *NCHHSTP social determinants of health: Frequently asked questions.* http://www.cdc.gov/nchhstp/socialdeterminants/faq.html (accessed September 22, 2016).

CMA (Canadian Medical Association). 2013. *Health equity and the social determinants of health: A role for the medical profession.* Ottawa, ON: Canadian Medical Association.

Cohen, J. J., B. A. Gabriel, and C. Terrell. 2002. The case for diversity in the health care workforce. *Health Affairs* 21:90-102.

COGME (Council on Graduate Medical Education). 1998. *Physician distribution and health care challenges in rural and inner-city areas, tenth report.* Washington, DC: COGME.

CORDIS (Community Research and Development Information Service). 2015. *Indepth training and research centres of excellence.* http://cordis.europa.eu/project/rcn/101109_en.html (accessed February 1, 2016).

Dapremont, J. A. 2012. A review of minority recruitment and retention models implemented in undergraduate nursing programs. *Journal of Nursing Education and Practice* 3(2):112-119.

Dogra, N., S. Reitmanova, and O. Carter-Pokras. 2009. Twelve tips for teaching diversity and embedding it in the medical curriculum. *Medical Teacher* 31(11):990-993.

The Economist. 2012. *For richer, for poorer.* http://www.economist.com/node/21564414 (accessed September 22, 2016).

Elliott, C. M., O. Stransky, R. Negron, M. Bowlby, J. Lickiss, D. Dutt, N. Dasgupta, and P. Barbosa. 2013. Institutional barriers to diversity change work in higher education. *SAGE Open* 3(2):1-9.

Falkingham, J., M. Evandrou, and M. Lyons-Amos. 2012. *ESRC Centre for Population Change working paper, no. 24: Inequalities in child and maternal health outcomes in CEE and the CIS.* Southampton, England: Economic and Social Research Council Centre for Population Change.

Frenk, J., L. Chen, Z. A. Bhutta, J. Cohen, N. Crisp, T. Evans, H. Fineberg, P. Garcia, Y. Ke, P. Kelley, B. Kistnasamy, A. Meleis, D. Naylor, A. Pablos-Mendez, S. Reddy, S. Scrimshaw, J. Sepulveda, D. Serwadda, and H. Zurayk. 2010. Health professionals for a new century: Transforming education to strengthen health systems in an interdependent world. *Lancet* 376(9756):1923-1958.

Gijón-Sánchez, M.-T., S. Pinzón-Pulido, R.-L. Kolehmainen-Aitken, J. Weekers, D. L. Acuña, R. Benedict, and M.-J. Peiro. 2010. Better health for all in Europe: Developing a migrant sensitive health workforce. *Eurohealth* 16(1):17.

Government of Canada. 2015. *Rio political declaration on social determinants of health: A snapshot of Canadian actions 2015.* http://www.healthycanadians.gc.ca/publications/ science-research-sciences-recherches/rio/index-eng.php (accessed February 1, 2016).

Grumbach, K., and R. Mendoza. 2008. Disparities in human resources: Addressing the lack of diversity in the health professions. *Health Affairs (Millwood)* 27(2):413-422.

Haney, T. J. 2015. Factory to faculty: Socioeconomic difference and the educational experiences of university professors. *Canadian Review of Sociology/Revue Canadienne de Sociologie* 52(2):160-186.

HHS (U.S. Department of Health and Human Services). 2010. *Healthy People 2020.* Washington, DC: HHS. http://www.healthypeople.gov/sites/default/files/HP2020_brochure_ with_LHI_508_FNL.pdf (accessed January 11, 2016).

HHS. 2016a. *Healthypeople.gov: Disparities.* http://www.healthypeople.gov/2020/about/ foundation-health-measures/Disparities (accessed January 28, 2016).

HHS. 2016b. *Healthypeople.gov: Determinants of health.* http://www.healthypeople.gov/2020/ about/foundation-health-measures/Determinants-of-Health (accessed January 11, 2016).

HHS. 2016c. *Healthypeople.gov: Social determinants of health.* http://www.healthypeople. gov/2020/topics-objectives/topic/social-determinants-health (accessed February 1, 2016).

HRSA (Health Resources and Services Administration). 2006. *The rationale for diversity in the health professions: A review of the evidence* Washington, DC: HRSA.

IFMSA (International Federation of Medical Students' Associations). 2014. *IFMSA policy statement: Health equity and the social determinants of health.* http://ifmsa.org/ wp-content/uploads/2015/05/SecGen_2014AM_PS_Health_Equity_and_the_Social_ Determinants_of_Health.pdf (accessed February 1, 2016).

Jones, C. P., C. Y. Jones, G. S. Perry, G. Barclay, and C. A. Jones. 2009. Addressing the social determinants of children's health: A cliff analogy. *Journal of Health Care for the Poor and Underserved* 20(Suppl. 4):1-12.

Ko, M., K. C. Heslin, R. A. Edelstein, and K. Grumbach. 2007. The role of medical education in reducing health care disparities: The first ten years of the UCLA/Drew Medical Education Program. *Journal of General Internal Medicine* 22(5):625-631.

Link, B. G., and J. Phelan. 1995. Social conditions as fundamental causes of disease. *Journal of Health and Social Behavior* Spec. No. 80-94.

Lomazzi, M., C. Jenkins, and B. Borisch. 2016. Global public health today: Connecting the dots. *Global Health Action* 9:28772.

MA4Health (Measurement and Accountability for Results in Health). 2015. *Measurement and Accountability for Results in Health: A common agenda for the post-2015 era.* http:// ma4health.hsaccess.org/goal-objectives (accessed February 1, 2016).

Markwick, A., Z. Ansari, M. Sullivan, L. Parsons, and J. McNeil. 2014. Inequalities in the social determinants of health of Aboriginal and Torres Strait Islander people: A cross-sectional population-based study in the Australian state of Victoria. *International Journal for Equity in Health* 13:91.

Marmot, M. 2005. Social determinants of health inequalities. *Lancet* 365(9464):1099-1104.

Marmot, M., and J. J. Allen. 2014. Social determinants of health equity. *American Journal of Public Health* 104(Suppl. 4):S517-S519.

Marmot, M., A. Pellegrini Filho, J. Vega, O. Solar, and K. Fortune. 2013. Action on social determinants of health in the Americas. *Revista Panamericana de Salud Pública* 34(6):379-384.

McGinnis, J. M., and W. H. Foege. 1993. Actual causes of death in the United States. *Journal of the American Medical Association* 270(18):2207-2212.

McGinnis, J. M., P. Williams-Russo, and J. R. Knickman. 2002. The case for more active policy attention to health promotion. *Health Affairs (Millwood)* 21(2):78-93.

Mihalynuk, T. V., P. Soule Odegard, R. Kang, M. Kedzierski, and N. Johnson Crowley. 2007. Partnering to enhance interprofessional service-learning innovations and addictions recovery. *Education for Health (Abingdon, England)* 20(3):92.

Moscrop, A. 2012. Health inequalities in primary care: Time to face justice. *The British Journal of General Practice* 62(601):428-429.

Mulé, N. J., L. E. Ross, B. Deeprose, B. E. Jackson, A. Daley, A. Travers, and D. Moore. 2009. Promoting LGBT health and wellbeing through inclusive policy development. *International Journal for Equity in Health* 8:18.

Nivet, M. A., and A. Berlin. 2014. Workforce diversity and community-responsive health-care institutions. *Public Health Reports* 129(Suppl. 2):15-18.

OECD (Organisation for Economic Co-operation and Development), Eurostat, and WHO-Europe. 2015. *Joint data collection on non-monetary health care statistics: Joint questionnaire 2015. Guidelines for completing the OECD/Eurostat/WHO-Europe questionnaire 2015.* http://www.oecd.org/statistics/data-collection/Health%20Data%20-%20 Guidelines%202.pdf (accessed September 22, 2016).

Paradies, Y., J. Ben, N. Denson, A. Elias, N. Priest, A. Pieterse, A. Gupta, M. Kelaher, and G. Gee. 2015. Racism as a determinant of health: A systematic review and meta-analysis. *PLoS ONE* 10(9):e0138511.

Phillips, J. M., and B. Malone. 2014. Increasing racial/ethnic diversity in nursing to reduce health disparities and achieve health equity. *Public Health Reports* 129(Suppl. 2):45-50.

Price, E. G., A. Gozu, D. E. Kern, N. R. Powe, G. S. Wand, S. Golden, and L. A. Cooper. 2005. The role of cultural diversity climate in recruitment, promotion, and retention of faculty in academic medicine. *Journal of General Internal Medicine* 20(7):565-571.

Price, E. G., N. R. Powe, D. E. Kern, S. H. Golden, G. S. Wand, and L. A. Cooper. 2009. Improving the diversity climate in academic medicine: Faculty perceptions as a catalyst for institutional change. *Academic Medicine* 84(1):95-105.

Reading, C., and F. Wien. 2009. *Health inequalities and social determinants of Aboriginal peoples' health.* Prince George, BC: National Collaborating Centre for Aboriginal Health.

RWJF (Robert Wood Johnson Foundation). 2008. *Overcoming obstacles to health: Report from the Robert Wood Johnson Foundation to the Commission to Build a Healthier America.* Princeton, NJ: RWJF.

Solar, O., and A. Irwin. 2010. *A conceptual framework for action on the social determinants of health. Social determinants of health discussion paper 2 (policy and practice).* Geneva, Switzerland: WHO. http://www.who.int/sdhconference/resources/Conceptualframework foractiononSDH_eng.pdf (accessed September 22, 2016).

UNDP (United Nations Development Programme). 2013. *Discussion paper: Addressing the social determinants of noncommunicable diseases.* New York: UNDP.

United Nations. 2015. *Transforming our world: The 2030 agenda for sustainable development.* https://sustainabledevelopment.un.org/post2015/transformingourworld (accessed September 22, 2016).

WHO (World Health Organization). 2006. *The World Health Report 2006: Working together for health.* Geneva, Switzerland: WHO.

WHO. 2008. *Closing the gap in a generation: Health equity through action on the social determinants of health, final report.* Geneva, Switzerland: WHO Commission on Social Determinants of Health.

WHO. 2009. *Handbook on monitoring and evaluation of human resources for health: With special applications for low- and middle-income countries.* Geneva, Switzerland: WHO.

WHO. 2011. *Rio political declaration on social determinants of health.* Adopted at the World Conference on the Social Determinants of Health, Rio de Janeiro, Brazil. Geneva, Switzerland: WHO. http://www.who.int/sdhconference/declaration/Rio_political_declaration.pdf?ua=1 (accessed September 22, 2016).

WHO. 2013a. *A universal truth: No health without a workforce.* Geneva, Switzerland: WHO.

WHO. 2013b. Funding, flexible management needed for Brazil's health worker gaps. *Bulletin of the World Health Organization* 91(11):797-896.

WHO. 2014. *Review of social determinants and the health divide in the WHO European region: Final report.* Copenhagen, Denmark: WHO.

WHO. 2015a. *Health in all policies: Training manual.* Geneva, Switzerland: WHO.

WHO. 2015b. *Human resources for health information system: Minimum data set for health workforce registry.* Geneva, Switzerland: WHO.

WHO. 2016a. *Social determinants of health.* http://www.who.int/topics/social_determinants/en (accessed February 2, 2016).

WHO. 2016b. *Social determinants of health.* http://www.who.int/social_determinants/action_sdh/en (accessed February 1, 2016).

WHPA (World Health Professions Alliance). 2010. *WHPA statement on non-communicable diseases and social determinants of health.* Ferney Voltaire, France: WHPA.

Williams, D. R. 1999. Race, socioeconomic status, and health. The added effects of racism and discrimination. *Annals of the New York Academy of Sciences* 896:173-188.

Wirth, M., E. Delamonica, E. Sacks, D. Balk, A. Storeygard, and A. Minujin. 2006. *Monitoring health equity in the MDGS: A practical guide.* Palisades, NY: Center for International Earth Science Information Network.

WKKF (W.K. Kellogg Foundation). 2016. *Grants.* http://www.wkkf.org/grants (accessed July 20, 2016).

2

Educating Health Professionals to Address the Social Determinants of Health in and with Communities

SUMMARY

This chapter reviews individual efforts to address the social determinants of health that informed the development of the committee's framework and recommendations presented in Chapter 4. This review goes beyond the published literature to include additional examples that have not been published in peer-reviewed journals so as to provide a broader view of the activities being used to educate health professionals in the social determinants of health across the educational spectrum. In addition, this chapter calls attention to important differences between the work of health care providers, who are trained to impact individual health outcomes, and public health workers, who are trained to impact the health of populations. Over the years, efforts have been made to bridge these two perspectives. This chapter describes one such model—community-oriented primary care—as well as long-standing networks and partnerships and lessons learned about educating health professionals to understand the broader construct of health systems. Also described is problem-based learning, a tool for offering innovative education that can develop critical thinking and drive a desire for continued learning about the social determinants of health. Discussed as well are workforce development and continuing professional development.

HISTORICAL PERSPECTIVE

Many of the concepts behind community-engaged learning, problem-based learning, and community-oriented education grew out of the work of Sidney and Emily Kark (Gofin, 2006). As early as 1940, the Karks began blending community engagement with public health practice and primary care in an impoverished, rural province of South Africa in what they called "community-oriented primary care" (Mullan and Epstein, 2002). According to Geiger (2002), the Karks understood that "social, economic, and environmental circumstances are the most powerful determinants of population health status" (p. 1713). Their ideas and theories spread around the globe, influencing health care delivery in such places as Jerusalem, the Republic of South Africa, the United Kingdom, and the United States (Geiger, 1993, 2002; Mullan and Epstein, 2002). They also led to numerous education and training programs in Chile, Cuba, Egypt, Europe, India, Israel, the Philippines, South Africa, Sudan, and the United States (Risley et al., 1989; THEnet, 2015a,b). While those educational initiatives did not explicitly reference the social determinants of health, because they predated the origin of that construct, they did involve education in communities that was focused on the social and environmental causes of ill health (Magzoub et al., 1992; Risley et al., 1989).

The lack of explicit recognition of the term "social determinants of health" is not uncommon. For example, mission statements, strategic documents, and curricula from the field of social work typically emphasize "social justice" despite having a strong focus on interventions addressing the social determinants of health (CASW, n.d.; Craig et al., 2013). Of course, the opposite is also true. Some programs that tout learning activities addressing the social determinants of health in reality provide only segments of a curriculum—for example, teaching statistics about health disparities in isolation, offering community service projects with no contextual framing or opportunities for reflection, providing only classroom education with no experiential component, and offering educational opportunities for learning about health disparities only in clinical (not community) settings (Cené et al., 2010; Chokshi, 2010). While potentially valuable, no one such activity performed in isolation provides learners a full understanding of how the different components of a health system are integrated and thus how the learner's role fits with others in the wider health system. Without such an orientation, understanding and acting on the social determinants of health in partnership with others will prove difficult if not impossible.

Networks and Partnerships

In 1979, leaders of mainly small pilot medical models of community-oriented education gathered for the first time in Kingston, Jamaica, to share their work, ideas, and aspirations (The Network, 2004, 2014a). At this meeting, participants agreed to form a group of interconnected health science innovation educators in what came to be known as The Network (Kantrowitz et al., 1987). Years later, The Network joined with another World Health Organization (WHO) initiative called Towards Unity for Health (TUFH) to create what is now known as The Network: Towards Unity for Health (also known as The Network). This nongovernmental organization advocates for community-engaged health professional education through local and international actions, partnerships, and sharing of ideas and expertise (The Network, 2014b).

Other groups have since undertaken similar efforts to make health professional education more responsive and relevant to societal needs (Richards, 2001). One such entity is the Training for Health Equity Network (THEnet), a "growing global movement committed to achieving health equity through health professions education, research and service that is responsive to the priority needs of communities" (THEnet, 2015c). Community engagement is an important component of all the work done by THEnet and its member schools, and partnerships with communities are part of THEnet's development, implementation, and evaluation efforts (THEnet, 2015c). Its member schools are from Australia, Belgium, Canada, Cuba, Nepal, the Philippines, South Africa, Sudan, and the United States (THEnet, 2015b).

The nonprofit membership organization Community-Campus Partnerships for Health (CCPH) is another effort to address the social determinants of health (CCPH, n.d.). Established in 1997, its focus is on promoting health equity and social justice. CCPH connects communities and campuses in the United States and in Canada to improve the health of communities through service learning, community-based participatory research, broad-based coalitions, and other partnership strategies (CCPH, 2007).

The U.S. government is currently developing Healthy People 2020. The Healthy People 2020 and related websites highlight the importance of addressing the social determinants of health and including prevention and population health content in health professionals' education (APTR, 2016; HHS, 2016a,b,c). This effort has led to numerous online educational resources for students and health professionals to learn how to reach national health goals (HHS, 2016d). Another U.S.-based initiative is working through the Association of Academic Health Centers to raise awareness and build partnerships for a more coordinated response to addressing the social determinants of health (AAHC, 2015; Wartman, 2010; Wartman and Steinberg, 2011).

Lessons Learned

Between 1998 and 2000, The Network identified nine health professional education programs deemed exemplary (Richards, 2001). Criteria for inclusion were based on demonstration of the following educational components:

- commitment to multidisciplinary and community-based education,
- longitudinal community placements,
- formal linkages with government entities, and
- a structured approach to community participation.

Each of the nine schools (in Chile, Cuba, Egypt, India, the Philippines, South Africa, Sudan, Sweden, and the United States) was visited by one of The Network's researchers. In his overall review of the programs, Richards (2001) identifies common features and shared dilemmas among programs:

- All of the exemplars provided a variety of community-based learning experiences, and most used a problem-based learning approach.
- While the different schools required similar competencies and knowledge for graduation, the local context drove the individual student activities.
- Learning to work collaboratively with other professionals and professions was deemed essential.
- All of the programs emphasized the relationship between individual and population health, which typically included a local socioeconomic perspective.
- Interventions and strategies are meaningless unless they match local needs and conditions.
- Learning to advocate for patients and the community is an important aspect of career development, particularly as it relates to public policy.
- Institutionalization of innovative reforms is slow and sometimes never realized, despite 5-10 years of sustained involvement by deans and distinguished faculty members.

Fourteen years later, Strasser and colleagues (2015) drew lessons from rural, community-engaged medical schools in Australia, Canada, and the Philippines. They concluded that community engagement must be sensitive to local variations; community leaders need to be pursuaded of the value of engaging with universities through open and honest dialogue; and stronger partnerships will develop if differences between partners are viewed as complementary assets rather than challenges (Strasser et al., 2015). The sustainability of such a program will depend heavily on the success of the local partnership, although success also will depend on the national and sub-national context in which a program functions (Coffman and Henderson, 2001; Loh et al., 2013; Supe and Burdick, 2006).

Additional lessons can be learned from countries with national health systems that align education with health service delivery. In Brazil, for example, health professional education and the health workforce are shared responsibilities of the Ministry of Education and the Brazilian Unified Health System (Sistema Único de Saúde [SUS]), which guarantees universal and free health care coverage for all. These two bodies work together through the Interministerial Committee for Education and Health Labour Management, which was established in 2007 (WHO, 2013a). Much of their work is based on the integration of teaching and service through multi-disciplinary teams and has led to innovations in community-based education and explicit use of community health agents to establish linkages with care and wellness efforts (Bollela et al., 2015; Macinko and Harris, 2015). One education example, known as the Education Program for Health Work (PET Health), is the Ministry of Health strategy for promoting teaching-service-community integration by creating working groups of teachers, undergraduate students, and health professionals for interprofessional education and practice (Bollela et al., 2015). Faculty supervise undergraduate students working in primary health care in Family Health Units. These units are part of Brazil's Family Health Strategy (previously called the Family Health Program), which is aimed at providing a range of health care services to families in their homes, at clinics, and in hospitals (WHO, 2008). Rapid expansion of the Family Health Strategy led to shortages of health professionals. This gap was filled through the recruitment of almost 15,000 physicians, primarily from Cuba. Studies on the strategy's expansion have shown improved children's health and reduced infant mortality, as well as associations with diminished mortality from cardio- and cerebrovascular events, reductions in hospital admissions, and fewer rates of complications from diabetes (Macinko and Harris, 2015; Paim et al., 2011; Rasella et al., 2014; Rocha and Soares, 2010).

Not without difficulties, Brazil has been pursuing this path for several decades. Substantial investments have been made to change the curricula of medical, dental, and nursing schools, leading them to integrate students into the public Unified Health System and making them more responsive to the needs of the communities they serve, rather than just individual patients (Bollela et al., 2015; Ferreira et al., 2007). National guidelines have been revamped and principles adopted that are conducive to greater emphasis on the social determinants of health and health inequalities.

Cuba is another country with a strong national health system that relies heavily on primary care providers who are trained in rural settings with community service as a requirement (Morales Idel et al., 2008). To align education with health and workforce needs, the Cuban Ministries of Education, Higher Education, and Public Health all take responsibility for training health professionals. The academic requirements are set by the Ministries of Health and Education, while the Ministry of Public Health sets up and maintains the actual training for the university-level health science professions (Morales Idel et al., 2008). This public health orientation has led to curriculum reform as the Ministry of Public Health has sought to balance Cuba's changing population health profile with needed human resources for health to meet the health system's staffing needs. These efforts have included identifying and enrolling in medical schools qualified students from underserved populations who are expected to return to their community following graduation (Keck and Reed, 2012).

Despite these two examples, alignment between the education and health sectors and between the health system and the needs of communities remains weak in most countries (Frenk et al., 2010). Greater alignment would support and empower communities, the health workforce, and educators to work together in an equal partnership to address the social determinants of health, recognizing that context and circumstances will determine the shape, form, and nature of these partnerships (Chiang et al., 2015; WHO, 2013b).

ANALYZING THE EVIDENCE BASE

Searching the literature for impact studies of experiential, community-based, or community-engaged learning activities that specifically identify the social determinants of health as an impact measure presents numerous difficulties. Publication biases exist toward developed, English-speaking countries, and terminology differs among countries and programs. If the term "social determinants of health" is not used in an article, for example, the search will not identify that article. Articles that will be missed include those addressing programs established before the term "social determinants of health" was coined. As a result, some published programs and activities may have been missed during the literature review conducted for the present study. However, because the statement of task for this study (see Box 1-1 in Chapter 1) refers specifically to the social determinants of health, the search conducted for the background paper commissioned by the committee was narrowed accordingly, and 33 relevant papers were identified (see Appendix A for more detail). What is remarkable about the findings of this review is how varied these programs were and how few of their evaluations looked beyond learning outcomes. In addition, the vast majority of the programs relied on self-reported information from the learners themselves. While interesting, these reported findings do not help determine whether the educational intervention or activity impacted the social determinants of health, improved the health or well-being of the community, or should be considered for diffusion or scale-up.

The lack of analysis of outcomes with respect to improving the health and well-being of communities and their members is due to a multitude of research and resource issues (Art et al., 2007). Identifying linkages between education and health outcomes is time-consuming and requires specific expertise to produce accurate findings. Also, confounding factors related to community movement and migration as well as project funding can alter the results in ways that make accurate data analysis impossible (Art et al., 2007). Despite these challenges, efforts have been made to determine the impacts of service-learning and community-based educational interventions. Most of the published work in this area either is descriptive or emphasizes learning outcomes of uniprofessional education (Dongre et al., 2010; Essa-Hadad et al., 2015; Klein and Vaughn, 2010; O'Brien et al., 2014; Rebholz et al., 2013; Whelan and Black, 2007), although there are some examples describing interprofessional community-based education and learning outcomes (Art et al., 2007; Bainbridge et al., 2014; Mihalynuk et al., 2007). One such example, described in Box 2-1, is an interprofessional, longitudinal, community-engaged curriculum recently established at Florida International University's Herbert Wertheim College of Medicine. The purpose of the curriculum is to educate students in and with communities on the social determinants of health. After 1 year of home visits provided in the context of medical and health education interventions, analyses indicate favorable short-term and intermediate impacts on health, cost savings, and efficacy (Rock et al., 2014).

Other examples drawn from medicine, nursing, dentistry, and public health education have been implemented with the intent of impacting health systems, as well as the chronic disease profiles of communities and their members (Ferreira et al., 2007; Lipman et al., 2011; Ross et al., 2014; Sabo et al., 2015). Examples from social work education include efforts to build community partnerships (Mokuau et al., 2008; Wertheimer et al., 2004). In particular, Mokuau and colleagues (2008) and others show how the application of principles of community-based participatory research that align with cultural values can impact health inequities through social change (Braun et al., 2006; Kaholokula et al., 2013; Mokuau et al., 2008). In dental education, a study on the financial implications of placing students in community clinics found that dental students make a significant contribution to clinic productivity and finances (Le et al., 2011).

Some university programs have sought to emulate the success of agriculture extension programs in reaching local communities. The University of Kentucky's Health Education through Extension Leadership program is a partnership between the College of Public Health and the College of

---

BOX 2-1
Herbert Wertheim College of Medicine
Curriculum on Social Determinants of Health

Florida International University's (FIU's) Herbert Wertheim College of Medicine (HWCOM) is an innovative twenty-first-century medical school founded in 2006. Its unique doctor of medicine degree curriculum emphasizes the social determinants of health—both in the traditional classroom setting and in the community classroom—through team-based, household-centered care. The college's Green Family Foundation Neighborhood Health Education Learning Program (NeighborhoodHELP™) provides students with longitudinal, interprofessional, service-learning experiences that allow students to translate classroom learning into practical application throughout the curriculum. The program addresses health disparities through reflection on social determinants of health in urban underserved households. A strong university–community partnership is at the core of this novel approach.

HWCOM faculty and staff develop relationships with local community agencies, forging partnerships to influence policy and improve population health. These community partners identify underserved households and refer them to NeighborhoodHELP™. Outreach teams visit each referred household to assess members' needs and eligibility for services. Engaging communities through this structure has resulted in a sustained flow of households participating in the program, a comprehensive network of local resources, trusted relationships that inform development of the curriculum, and continuity of household-centered care for participants who previously relied solely on emergency departments or America's "safety net" for health care services.

Agriculture and its Cooperative Extension Service. The program focuses on reducing Kentucky's chronic disease rates through dissemination of health and wellness information on preventable risk factors (Riley, 2008). At the University of New Mexico Health Sciences Center (UNMHSC), honest and at times disheartening conversations with rural community leaders led to the establishment of a statewide Health Extension Rural Office (HERO) program (Kaufman et al., 2010, 2015). The program focuses on community-derived health priorities within the university's mission areas of education, clinical service, and research. It is run through the university's Office of the Vice President for Community Health, which collaborates with the New Mexico Department of Health to develop county health report cards. The report cards provide data on leading causes of morbidity and mortality, as well as information on the health workforce, community planning priorities, and the center's programs. HERO agents use the report cards to track the responsiveness and effectiveness of UNMHSC programs in addressing community health needs. One diabetes education program

The HWCOM curriculum is built on study in five major strands: human biology; disease, illness, and injury; clinical medicine; professional development; and medicine and society. Within the medicine and society strand, a series of Community-Engaged Physician courses is horizontally and vertically integrated across all periods and incorporates the Healthy People 2020 social determinants of health framework and leading health indicators. Related curricula include ethics, cultural humility, social and cultural influences on health, interprofessional communication and teamwork, household-centered care, and population health. In addition to situated learning during household visits, educational modalities include active learning sessions, small-group activities, student presentations, classroom discussions, didactic or panel presentations, role play, concept mapping, and reflective writing.

Interprofessional teams of FIU faculty with expertise in primary care (including family medicine, internal medicine, and pediatrics), psychiatry, public health, ethics, anthropology, law, social work, nursing, and education supervise student teams generally comprising medical, nursing, and social work students. Students enrolled in the college's new physician assistant studies program will begin participating in 2016. Students conduct biopsychosocial assessments; provide educational, primary care, social, and behavioral services; and assist household members in navigating and managing health and social services. HWCOM's focus on addressing social determinants of health aims to reduce health disparities, foster community engagement, and transform the health of patients and communities.

SOURCE: Based on a presentation by Onelia G. Lage, M.D., FAAP, Florida International University, at the committee's open session on September 15, 2015.

led to a significant drop in HbA_{1C} levels of Hispanic patients with diabetes (Kaufman et al., 2010).

Numerous publications have identified a need for public health schools and institutes to educate learners more actively in policy and advocacy, given the important role of policy change in population health (Caira et al., 2003; Fleming et al., 2009; Hearne, 2008; Hines and Jernigan, 2012; Mirzoev et al., 2014; Pandey et al., 2012). However, information on courses designed to educate health professional learners about translating public health science into policy action is incomplete and limited (Pandey et al., 2012). Longest and Huber (2010, p. 50) describe key steps that public health schools can take to enhance the capabilities of faculty with respect to influencing policy making: "(1) building infrastructures to support and facilitate this role, (2) teaching faculty members how to be more influential in the policy arena, and (3) aligning incentives and rewards for faculty who contribute to improved public health by influencing the formation and implementation of public health policy."

BUILDING A DIVERSE AND INCLUSIVE HEALTH WORKFORCE

One approach to building the diversity of the health workforce is through greater mixing of university and community representatives, potentially through work on pipeline initiatives (Nivet and Berlin, 2014; Snyder et al., 2015). In fact, numerous programs funded by the U.S. Department of Health and Human Services are aimed at broadening and enhancing pipeline programs designed to enable racial and ethnic minority and disadvantaged students to enter careers in the health professions and health sciences (HHS, 2009). While these programs hold great promise, enhanced information sharing across agencies and programs could improve coordination and sharing of lessons learned among agencies and programs (HHS, 2009).

In some ways, diversity is about collaboration—collaborating with different professions, institutions and programs, communities, populations, and sectors and with individuals from different backgrounds and cultures. It is the particular situation that dictates who will be engaged, and the players themselves will determine how best to manage the collaboration. For example, the Nursing Workforce Diversity Program of the Health Equity Academy at Duke University, described in Box 2-2, includes a partnership between program administrators and social workers. Involving social workers in its nursing program is one way the Academy helps to ensure the success of its students, who themselves may have experienced social and cultural challenges similar to those of the communities and patients they will be expected to interact with throughout their training and career.

Dogra and colleagues (2009) studied the potential for developing and delivering education in cultural diversity in medical schools across Canada, the United Kingdom, and the United States. They offer 12 suggestions for overcoming resistance through a multifaceted approach that entails integrating the subject into institutional policies, curriculum content, faculty development, and assessment. The first of the 12 suggestions is to "design a diversity and human rights education institutional policy" (p. 2) And while doing so would demonstrate leadership's interest in diversity, a gap will remain between diversity concepts and practice absent an environment of inclusivity of all students, faculty, and staff (Elliot et al., 2013; Haney, 2015).

Finally, engaging students in reviewing university policies on diversity and inclusivity exposes them to the concept of ineffective versus effective policy making. Similarly, students pursing clinical careers could be "trained to ask specific questions on rounds that frame individual patient encounters as windows into broader community health and policy issues" (Jacobsohn et al., 2008, abstract).

CONTINUING PROFESSIONAL DEVELOPMENT

Health professional education at the foundational education and training level is a small percentage of the overall learning that takes place throughout the career of a health professional. Therefore, continuing professional development represents an opportunity to build and maintain competencies in areas that, because of time and other constraints, could not be fully addressed during foundational education and training. These areas may include interprofessional education and community-engaged research.

One research-driven initiative began through the INDEPTH Network, based in Ghana. INDEPTH is an international network of demographic research institutions whose mission is to "harness the collective potential of the world's community-based longitudinal demographic surveillance initiatives in low and middle income countries to provide a better understanding of health and social issues and to encourage the application of this understanding to alleviate major health and social problems" (INDEPTH Network, n.d.). To this end, the network established INDEPTH Training and Research Centres of Excellence (INTRECs). These centers provide training related to the social determinants of health to INDEPTH researchers and enable information sharing with decision makers (INTREC, n.d.-a). INTREC training is divided into five blocks that are taught by faculty and specialists from Germany, Ghana, Indonesia, the Netherlands, South Africa, Sweden, and the United States:

Block 1: SDH [Social Determinants of Health] Framework, taught through an online course
Block 2: Methods to Study SDH, taught through mixed-methods workshops
Block 3: Data Analyses Workshop, taught through a workshop
Block 4: Communication Strategies, taught through an online seminar
Block 5: Sharing Results of the Training, done through an online forum (INTREC, n.d.-b)

Analysis of the baseline situation in each of the INTREC focus countries (Bangladesh, Ghana, India, Indonesia, South Africa, Tanzania, and Vietnam) is available through individually developed country reports (Addei et al., 2012; Kalage et al., 2012; Kekan et al., 2012; Maredza et al., 2012; Nahar et al., 2012; Phuong et al., 2012; Susilo et al., 2012). Each report follows a similar structure, which starts with a country analysis and ends with a series of actionable recommendations directed at government, nongovernmental organizations, and the INTREC itself. The analysis includes the following three primary areas:

BOX 2-2
Addressing Social Determinants of Health in a
Pre-Entry Immersion to Nursing Program to Cultivate
Success and Acclimation to the Nursing Profession

The Academy for Academic and Social Enrichment and Leadership Development for Health Equity (Health Equity Academy [HEA]), Nursing Workforce Diversity Program, Bureau of Health Workforce, Health Resources and Services Administration (HRSA), U.S. Department of Health and Human Services, represents an innovative conceptual multilevel/multidimensional approach to addressing the social determinants of health at the individual, social, and structural levels. The aim of this program is to increase the number of high-achieving/high-potential underrepresented minorities in nursing from economically disadvantaged backgrounds by achieving the following goals: (1) cultivate the next generation of minority nurse leaders who are committed to health equity; (2) strengthen the extent to which the Accelerated Bachelors of Science in Nursing (ABSN) curriculum prepares graduates who fully understand, appreciate, and are committed to addressing the interrelationships between and among social determinants of health, health access, and health disparities (health equity concepts); and (3) continue to advance as an academically and socially responsive center of excellence in the development of nursing workforce diversity.

HEA offers a summer pre-entry program to expand understanding of nursing as a career, promote the role of nursing and its interface with health equity concepts, continue to expand the health equity threads as adjunct experiences concurrent with enrollment in the ABSN program, and influence readiness for the ABSN program. HEA incorporates a focused assessment of individual-level social determinants of health in order to match financial, social, and academic interventions or strategies with need. These strategies include the following:

- A pre-entrance webinar informs participants of the infrastructure of the HEA program.
- An initial social determinants of health individual assessment is administered in order to identify individual social determinants that may be potential barriers to student success. Surveys are administered by the HEA social worker, and debrief is held afterward to address any potential distress caused by the sensitive nature of the questions. Surveys are reviewed and evaluated by the program director and social worker. Based on the HEA Scholars' responses, a Prescription for Success is created,

---

1. Collect information on training related to the social determinants of health currently taking place in the country.
2. Identify core issues related to the social determinants of health of concern for the country.
3. Gather and review relevant government policies and ongoing work of nongovernmental organizations in the country.

which incorporates individualized strategies and goals designed to enhance success. Individual and group sessions are held by the social work and project director quarterly to determine the efficacy of interventions, identify new barriers, and develop additional strategies if needed.

- Seminars are held to provide an understanding of individual and community social determinants of health, including *Introduction to the Pathophysiology of Disease Related to Social and Environmental Determinants of Health*. This seminar addresses social determinants of health as a precursor to alterations in biological processes that affect the body's dynamic equilibrium or homeostasis and the development of language to describe those alterations. The seminar also examines the pathophysiology, social determinants, risk factors, and clinical manifestations of common disease states, as evidenced by completion of critical thinking questions and clinical cases.
- The *Unnatural Causes* documentary series facilitates discussion of inequuities and influences on health outcomes.
- HEA Scholars complete a thorough assessment and windshield survey of the local community and present results in an open forum at the end of the immersion program.
- HEA Scholars participate in community engagement, such as working with local nonprofit agencies that serve underserved populations.
- Other components include journaling to encourage reflection and a budgeting program to minimize financial barriers.

Additional strategies to influence awareness, understanding, and commitment to health equity concepts among nursing faculty and communities of interest are provided through a Health Equity Colloquium. HEA collaborates with faculty to strengthen the ABSN curriculum by planning for the integration of health equity concepts throughout the curriculum and related learning experiences, and to implement the curriculum in a manner that will increase the capacity of all nurses to address health inequalities competently. The sense of diversity and inclusiveness of the academic and social milieu of the school is heightened by identifying and institutionalizing several evidence-based interventions congruent with environmental satisfaction among underrepresented minorities.

SOURCE: Based on a presentation by Brigit M. Carter, Ph.D., R.N., CCRN, Duke University School of Nursing, at the committee's open session on September 15, 2015.

Another example is the Society for Public Health Education's State Health Policy Institute (SHPI) curriculum, designed to educate U.S. state legislators and other professionals in the latest policies and research in chronic disease prevention and control (SOPHE, n.d.). Between 2009 and 2011, SHPI organized three courses and trained an elite corps of 40 health promotion policy experts on policy issues such as health education, nutrition, childhood obesity, eliminating health disparities, and tobacco prevention and education (SOPHE, n.d., preface).

Other programs and initiatives involve postdoctoral education and continuing professional development to promote professionals' learning in and with communities. Compared with data-driven projects, these activities often take a broader, more systems-based approach to learning and implementation (Beyond Flexner, n.d.; FAIMER, 2015; Kellogg Health Scholars, 2016; MEDICC, 2016). One example is the U.S. Robert Wood Johnson Foundation's Health & Society Scholars program, which targets individuals at the postdoctoral level at any stage in their career. Scholars receive 2 years of support to "investigate the connections among biological, behavioral, environmental, economic, and social determinants of health and develop, evaluate, and disseminate knowledge and interventions based upon these determinants" (De Milto, 2014). The program emphasizes collaboration and exchange across disciplines and sectors to address the determinants of population health and contribute to policy change. Another example is Medical Education Cooperation with Cuba's Community Partnerships for Health Equity. This program provides learning opporutnities for health profesionals to experience Cuba's community-engaged health and education system, and then adapt aspects of that model to improve health and health equity in communities in the United States (MEDICC, 2016). Communities in four underserved U.S. neighborhoods—South Los Angeles and Oakland, California; Albuquerque, New Mexico; and the Bronx, New York—have all benefited from a health profesional's initiative to learn about and take action on addressing the social determinants of health in and with their local communities.

REFERENCES

AAHC (Association of Academic Health Centers). 2015. *AAHC social determinants of health initiative: A toolkit for collaboration.* http://www.wherehealthbegins.org (accessed September 22, 2016).

Addei, S., Y. Blomstedt, M. Gyapong, M. Bangha, R. Preet, K. Hofman, and J. Kinsman. 2012. *INTREC: Ghana country report.* http://www.intrec.info/Country%20reports/INTREC%20-%20Ghana.pdf (accessed January 11, 2016).

APTR (Association for Prevention Teaching and Research). 2016. *APTR Healthy People Curriculum Task Force.* http://www.aptrweb.org/?page=HPC_Taskforce (accessed July 21, 2016).

Art, B., L. De Roo, and J. De Maeseneer. 2007. Towards Unity for Health utilising community-oriented primary care in education and practice. *Education for Health (Abingdon, England)* 20(2):74.

Bainbridge, L., S. Grossman, S. Dharamsi, J. Porter, and V. Wood. 2014. Engagement studios: Students and communities working to address the determinants of health. *Education for Health (Abingdon, England)* 27(1):78-82.

Beyond Flexner. n.d. *Welcome.* http://beyondflexner.org (accessed September 22, 2016).

Bollela, V. R., A. C. Germani, H. de Holanda Campos, and E. M. Amaral. 2015. *Community-based education for the health professions: Learning from the Brazilian experience.* São Paulo, Brazil: Pan American Health Organization.

Braun, K. L., J. U. Tsark, L. Santos, N. Aitaoto, and C. Chong. 2006. Building Native Hawaiian capacity in cancer research and programming. A legacy of 'Imi Hale. *Cancer* 107(8 Suppl.):2082-2090.

Caira, N. M., S. Lachenmayr, J. Sheinfeld, F. W. Goodhart, L. Cancialosi, and C. Lewis. 2003. The health educator's role in advocacy and policy: Principles, processes, programs, and partnerships. *Health Promotion Practice* 4(3):303-313.

Carter, B. 2015. *Academy for Academic and Social Enrichment & Leadership Development for Health Equity (Health Equity Academy).* Presented at the open session meeting of the Committee on Educating Health Professionals to Address the Social Determinants of Health. Washington, DC, September 15.

CASW (Canadian Association of Social Workers). n.d. *About CASW.* http://www.casw-acts.ca/en/about-casw (accessed September 22, 2016).

CCPH (Community-Campus Partnerships for Health). 2007. *Celebrating a decade of impact.* Seattle, WA: CCPH.

CCPH. n.d. *CCPH homepage.* https://ccph.memberclicks.net (accessed September 22, 2016).

Cené, C. W., M. E. Peek, E. Jacobs, and C. R. Horowitz. 2010. Community-based teaching about health disparities: Combining education, scholarship, and community service. *Journal of General Internal Medicine* 25(Suppl. 2):S130-S135.

Chiang, R. J., W. Meagher, and S. Slade. 2015. How the whole school, whole community, whole child model works: Creating greater alignment, integration, and collaboration between health and education. *Journal of School Health* 85(11):775-784.

Chokshi, D. A. 2010. Teaching about health disparities using a social determinants framework. *Journal of General Internal Medicine* 25(Suppl. 2):S182-S185.

Coffman, J., and T. Henderson. 2001. Public policies to promote community-based and interdisciplinary health professions education. *Education for Health (Abingdon, England)* 14(2):221-230.

Craig, S. L., R. Bejan, and B. Muskat. 2013. Making the invisible visible: Are health social workers addressing the social determinants of health? *Social Work in Health Care* 52(4):311-331.

De Milto, L. 2014. *Robert Wood Johnson Foundation Health & Society Scholars: An RWJF national program.* http://www.rwjf.org/en/library/research/2011/12/robert-wood-johnson-foundation-health---society-scholars.html (accessed February 5, 2016).

Dogra, N., S. Reitmanova, and O. Carter-Pokras. 2009. Twelve tips for teaching diversity and embedding it in the medical curriculum. *Medical Teacher* 31(11):990-993.

Dongre, A. R., P. R. Deshmukh, S. S. Gupta, and B. S. Garg. 2010. An evaluation of ROME camp: Forgotten innovation in medical education. *Education for Health (Abingdon, England)* 23(1):363.

Elliott, C. M., O. Stransky, R. Negron, M. Bowlby, J. Lickiss, D. Dutt, N. Dasgupta, and P. Barbosa. 2013. Institutional barriers to diversity change work in higher education. *SAGE Open* 3(2):1-9.

Essa-Hadad, J., D. Murdoch-Eaton, and M. C. Rudolf. 2015. What impact does community service learning have on medical students' appreciation of population health? *Public Health* 129(11):1444-1451.

FAIMER (Foundation for Advancement of International Medical Education and Research). 2015. *Education programs: Programs for health professionals.* Philadelphia, PA: FAIMER.

Ferreira, J. R., F. E. Campos, A. E. Haddad, and G. Cury. 2007. The challenge of improving health and medical care through undergraduate medical education "Pro-saude." *Education for Health (Abingdon, England)* 20(2):75.

Fleming, M. L., E. Parker, T. Gould, and M. Service. 2009. Educating the public health workforce: Issues and challenges. *Australia and New Zealand Health Policy* 6:1-8.

Frenk, J., L. Chen, Z. A. Bhutta, J. Cohen, N. Crisp, T. Evans, H. Fineberg, P. Garcia, Y. Ke, P. Kelley, B. Kistnasamy, A. Meleis, D. Naylor, A. Pablos-Mendez, S. Reddy, S. Scrimshaw, J. Sepulveda, D. Serwadda, and H. Zurayk. 2010. Health professionals for a new century: Transforming education to strengthen health systems in an interdependent world. *Lancet* 376(9756):1923-1958.

Geiger, H. J. 1993. Community-oriented primary care: The legacy of Sidney Kark. *American Journal of Public Health* 83(7):946-947.

Geiger, H. J. 2002. Community-oriented primary care: A path to community development. *American Journal of Public Health* 92(11):1713-1716.

Gofin, J. 2006. On "a practice of social medicine" by Sidney and Emily Kark. *Social Medicine* 1(2):107-115.

Haney, T. J. 2015. Factory to faculty: Socioeconomic difference and the educational experiences of university professors. *Canadian Review of Sociology/Revue Canadienne de Sociologie* 52(2):160-186.

Hearne, S. A. 2008. Practice-based teaching for health policy action and advocacy. *Public Health Reports* 123(Suppl. 2):65-70.

HHS (U.S. Department of Health and Human Services). 2009. *Pipeline programs to improve racial and ethnic diversity in the health professions: An inventory of federal programs, assessment of evaluation approaches, and critical review of the research literature.* Washington, DC: HHS.

HHS. 2016a. *HealthyPeople.gov: Educational and community-based programs.* http://www. healthypeople.gov/2020/topics-objectives/topic/educational-and-community-based-programs (accessed February 1, 2016).

HHS. 2016b. *HealthyPeople.gov: Social determinants of health.* http://www.healthypeople. gov/2020/topics-objectives/topic/social-determinants-health (accessed February 1, 2016).

HHS. 2016c. *Determinants of health.* https://www.healthypeople.gov/2020/about/foundation-health-measures/Determinants-of-Health (accessed July 21, 2016).

HHS. 2016d. *Healthy People eLearning.* https://www.healthypeople.gov/2020/tools-and-resources/Healthy-People-eLearning (accessed July 21, 2016).

Hines, A., and D. H. Jernigan. 2012. Developing a comprehensive curriculum for public health advocacy. *Health Promotion Practice* 13(6):733-737.

INDEPTH Network. n.d. *Vision, Mission & Strategic Objectives.* http://www.indepth-network. org/about-us/vision-mission-strategic-objectives-0 (accessed September 22, 2016).

INTREC (INDEPTH Training & Research Centres of Excellence). n.d.-a. *INTREC—INDEPTH Training & Research Centres of Excellence: Addressing Inequities and Social Determinants of Health in Asia & Africa.* http://www.intrec.info/intrecnew.html (accessed September 22, 2016).

INTREC. n.d.-b. *INTREC—INDEPTH Training & Research Centres of Excellence: Addressing Inequities and Social Determinants of Health in Asia & Africa. Training Program.* http://www.intrec.info/courses.html (accessed May 18, 2016).

Jacobsohn, V., M. DeArman, P. Moran, J. Cross, D. Dietz, R. Allen, S. Bachofer, L. Dow-Velarde, and A. Kaufman. 2008. Changing hospital policy from the wards: An introduction to health policy education. *Academic Medicine* 83(4):352-356.

Kaholokula, J. K., C. K. Townsend, A. Ige, K. Sinclair, M. K. Mau, A. Leake, D. M. Palakiko, S. R. Yoshimura, P. Kekauoha, and C. Hughes. 2013. Sociodemographic, behavioral, and biological variables related to weight loss in Native Hawaiians and other Pacific Islanders. *Obesity (Silver Spring)* 21(3):E196-E203.

Kalage, R., Y. Blomstedt, R. Preet, K. Hoffman, M. Bangha, and J. Kinsman. 2012. *INTREC: Tanzania country report.* http://www.intrec.info/Country%20reports/INTREC%20-%20 Tanzania.pdf (accessed January 11, 2016).

Kantrowitz, M., A. Kaufman, S. Mennin, T. Fulop, and J. J. Guilbert. 1987. *Innovative tracks at established institutions for the education of health personnel. An experimental approach to change relevant to health needs. WHO Offset Publication No. 101.* Geneva, Switzerland: WHO.

Kaufman, A., W. Powell, C. Alfero, M. Pacheco, H. Silverblatt, J. Anastasoff, F. Ronquillo, K. Lucero, E. Corriveau, B. Vanleit, D. Alverson, and A. Scott. 2010. Health extension in New Mexico: An academic health center and the social determinants of disease. *Annals of Family Medicine* 8(1):73-81.

Kaufman, A., P. B. Roth, R. S. Larson, N. Ridenour, L. S. Welage, V. Romero-Leggott, C. Nkouaga, K. Armitage, and K. L. McKinney. 2015. Vision 2020 measures University of New Mexico's success by health of its state. *American Journal of Preventive Medicine* 48(1):108-115.

Keck, C. W., and G. A. Reed. 2012. The curious case of Cuba. *American Journal of Public Health* 102(8):e13-e22.

Kekan, D., S. Juvekar, B. Wu, S. Padmawati, and J. Kinsman. 2012. *INTREC: India country report.* http://www.intrec.info/Country%20reports/INTREC%20-%20India.pdf (accessed January 11, 2016).

Kellogg Health Scholars. 2016. *Kellogg Health Scholars program.* http://www.kellogghealthscholars. org/about/history.php (accessed February 1, 2016).

Klein, M., and L. M. Vaughn. 2010. Teaching social determinants of child health in a pediatric advocacy rotation: Small intervention, big impact. *Medical Teacher* 32(9):754-759.

Lage, O. 2015. *Florida International University, Herbert Wertheim College of Medicine.* Presented at the open session meeting of the Committee on Educating Health Professionals to Address the Social Determinants of Health. Washington, DC, September 15.

Le, H., T. L. McGowan, and H. L. Bailit. 2011. Community-based dental education and community clinic finances. *Journal of Dental Education* 75(Suppl. 10):S48-S53.

Lipman, T. H., M. M. Schucker, S. J. Ratcliffe, T. Holmberg, S. Baier, and J. A. Deatrick. 2011. Diabetes risk factors in children: A partnership between nurse practitioner and high school students. *MCN: The American Journal of Maternal/Child Nursing* 36(1):56-62.

Loh, L. C., S. R. Friedman, and W. P. Burdick. 2013. Factors promoting sustainability of education innovations: A comparison of faculty perceptions and existing frameworks. *Education for Health (Abingdon, England)* 26(1):32-38.

Longest, B. B., and G. A. Huber. 2010. Schools of public health and the health of the public: Enhancing the capabilities of faculty to be influential in policymaking. *American Journal of Public Health* 100(1):49-53.

Macinko, J., and M. J. Harris. 2015. Brazil's family health strategy—delivering community-based primary care in a universal health system. *New England Journal of Medicine* 372(23):2177-2181.

Magzoub, M. M. A., D. O. Ahmed, and S. T. Taha. 1992. Eleven steps of community-based education as applied in Gezira Medical School. *Annals of Community Oriented Education* 5:11-17.

Maredza, M., K. Hofman, R. Preet, K. Kahn, M. Bangha, and J. Kinsman. 2012. *INTREC: South Africa country report.* http://www.intrec.info/Country%20reports/INTREC%20 -%20South%20Africa.pdf (accessed January 11, 2016).

MEDICC (Medical Education Cooperation with Cuba). 2016. *Community Partnerships for Health Equity (CPHE).* http://medicc.org/ns/?page_id=57 (accessed February 1, 2016).

Mihalynuk, T. V., P. Soule Odegard, R. Kang, M. Kedzierski, and N. Johnson Crowley. 2007. Partnering to enhance interprofessional service-learning innovations and addictions recovery. *Education for Health (Abingdon, England)* 20(3):92.

Mirzoev, T., G. Le, A. Green, M. Orgill, A. Komba, R. K. Esena, L. Nyapada, B. Uzochukwu, W. K. Amde, N. Nxumalo, and L. Gilson. 2014. Assessment of capacity for health policy and systems research and analysis in seven African universities: Results from the CHEPSAA project. *Health Policy Plan* 29(7):831-841.

Mokuau, N., C. V. Browne, K. L. Braun, and L. B. Choy. 2008. Using a community-based participatory approach to create a resource center for Native Hawaiian elders. *Education for Health (Abingdon, England)* 21(3):174.

Morales Idel, R., J. A. Fernandez, and F. Duran. 2008. Cuban medical education: Aiming for the six-star doctor. *MEDICC Review* 10(4):5-9.

Mullan, F., and L. Epstein. 2002. Community-oriented primary care: New relevance in a changing world. *American Journal of Public Health* 92(11):1748-1755.

Nahar, N., B. Wu, B. I. Kandarina, and J. Kinsman. 2012. *INTREC: Bangladesh country report.* http://www.intrec.info/Country%20reports/INTREC%20-%20Bangladesh.pdf (accessed January 11, 2016).

The Network. 2004. *The Network: Towards unity for health—newsletter.* https://issuu.com/thenetworktufh/docs/newsletter2004-01_0 (accessed February 2, 2016).

The Network. 2014a. *The Network: Towards unity for health—Prior Conferences.* http://thenetworktufh.org/conferences/prior-conferences (accessed May 16, 2016).

The Network. 2014b. *The Network: Towards unity for health—about us.* http://thenetworktufh.org/about (accessed May 16, 2016).

Nivet, M. A., and A. Berlin. 2014. Workforce diversity and community-responsive health-care institutions. *Public Health Reports* 129(Suppl. 2):15-18.

O'Brien, M. J., J. M. Garland, K. M. Murphy, S. J. Shuman, R. C. Whitaker, and S. C. Larson. 2014. Training medical students in the social determinants of health: The Health Scholars Program at Puentes de Salud. *Advances in Medical Education and Practice* 5:307-314.

Paim, J., C. Travassos, C. Almeida, L. Bahia, and J. Macinko. 2011. The Brazilian health system: History, advances, and challenges. *Lancet* 377(9779):1778-1797.

Pandey, A., K. Sharma, H. Hasan, and S. P. Zodpey. 2012. Emerging need for health policy teaching in India. *Indian Journal of Public Health* 56(3):210-213.

Phuong, T. B., T. P. Thao, M. Eriksson, R. Preet, L. Trisnantoro, and J. Kinsman. 2012. *INTREC: Vietnam country report.* http://www.intrec.info/Country%20reports/INTREC%20-%20Vietnam.pdf (accessed January 11, 2016).

Rasella, D., M. O. Harhay, M. L. Pamponet, R. Aquino, and M. L. Barreto. 2014. Impact of primary health care on mortality from heart and cerebrovascular diseases in Brazil: A nationwide analysis of longitudinal data. *BMJ* 349:g4014.

Rebholz, C. M., M. W. Macomber, M. D. Althoff, M. Garstka, A. Pogribny, A. Rosencrans, S. Selzer, and B. Springgate. 2013. Integrated models of education and service involving community-based health care for underserved populations: Tulane student-run free clinics. *Southern Medical Journal* 106(3):217-223.

Richards, R. W. 2001. Best practices in community-oriented health professions education: International exemplars. *Education for Health (Abingdon, England)* 14(3):357-365.

Riley, P. 2008. Collaboration for prevention of chronic disease in Kentucky: The Health Education through Extension Leaders (HEEL) program. *Nursing Clinics of North America* 43(3):vii, 329-340.

Risley, B., R. P. Foley, Z. M. Nooman, R. W. Richards, E. Ezzat, and F. Maklady. 1989. A collaboration between two innovative medical education programmes in Egypt and the United States. *Medical Education* 23(4):333-338.

Rocha, R., and R. R. Soares. 2010. Evaluating the impact of community-based health interventions: Evidence from Brazil's family health program. *Health Economics* 19(Suppl.):126-158.

Rock, J. A., J. M. Acuna, J. M. Lozano, I. L. Martinez, P. J. Greer, Jr., D. R. Brown, L. Brewster, and J. L. Simpson. 2014. Impact of an academic-community partnership in medical education on community health: Evaluation of a novel student-based home visitation program. *Southern Medical Journal* 107(4):203-211.

Ross, S. J., R. Preston, I. C. Lindemann, M. C. Matte, R. Samson, F. D. Tandinco, S. L. Larkins, B. Palsdottir, and A. J. Neusy. 2014. The training for health equity network evaluation framework: A pilot study at five health professional schools. *Education for Health (Abingdon, England)* 27(2):116-126.

Sabo, S., J. de Zapien, N. Teufel-Shone, C. Rosales, L. Bergsma, and D. Taren. 2015. Service learning: A vehicle for building health equity and eliminating health disparities. *American Journal of Public Health* 105(Suppl. 1):S38-S43.

Snyder, C. R., B. Stover, S. M. Skillman, and B. K. Frogner. 2015. *Facilitating racial and ethnic diversity in the health workforce.* Seattle, WA: University of Washington Health Workforce Research Center on Allied Health.

SOPHE (Society for Public Health Education). n.d. *Chronic disease policy: Guide to effectively educating state and local policymakers.* http://www.sophe.org/CDP/Ed_Policymakers_Guide.cfm (accessed February 2, 2016).

Strasser, R., P. Worley, F. Cristobal, D. C. Marsh, S. Berry, S. Strasser, and R. Ellaway. 2015. Putting communities in the driver's seat: The realities of community-engaged medical education. *Academic Medicine* 90(11):1466-1470.

Supe, A., and W. P. Burdick. 2006. Challenges and issues in medical education in India. *Academic Medicine* 81(12):1076-1080.

Susilo, D., M. Eriksson, R. Preet, L. Trisnantoro, S. Padmawati, B. I. Kandarina, and J. Kinsman. 2012. *INTREC: Indonesia country report.* http://www.intrec.info/Country%20reports/INTREC%20-%20Indonesia.pdf (accessed January 11, 2016).

THEnet (The Training for Health Equity Network). 2015a. *Sudan: University of Gezira—Faculty of Medicine (FMUG).* http://thenetcommunity.org/thenet-schools/sudan (accessed September 22, 2016).

THEnet. 2015b. *THEnet schools: Overview.* http://thenetcommunity.org/thenet-schools (accessed September 22, 2016).

THEnet. 2015c. *Our vision, mission, values, and approach.* http://thenetcommunity.org/our-vision-mission-values-approach (accessed May 16, 2016).

Wartman, S. A. 2010. *The compelling value proposition of academic health centers.* Washington, DC: Association of Academic Health Centers.

Wartman, S. A., and M. J. Steinberg. 2011. The role of academic health centers in addressing social responsibility. *Medical Teacher* 33(8):638-642.

Wertheimer, M., E. Beck, F. Brooks, and J. Wolk. 2004. Community partnerships: An innovative model of social work education and practice. *Journal of Community Practice* 12(3/4):123-140.

Whelan, A. K., and D. Black. 2007. Integrating public health and medicine: First steps in a new curriculum. *Education for Health (Abingdon, England)* 20(3):122.

WHO (World Health Organization). 2008. Flawed but fair: Brazil's health system reaches out to the poor. *Bulletin of the World Health Organization* 86(4):241-320.

WHO. 2013a. Funding, flexible management needed for Brazil's health worker gaps. *Bulletin of the World Health Organization* 91(11):797-896.

WHO. 2013b. *Transforming and scaling up health professionals' education and training: World Health Organization guidelines 2013.* Geneva, Switzerland: WHO.

3

Frameworks for Addressing the Social Determinants of Health

SUMMARY

This chapter describes the frameworks the committee reviewed in developing a single unified framework for educating health professionals in the social determinants of health. All of these ten frameworks have unique perspectives that can be grouped into several categories. The first two discussed in this chapter put the community in charge of taking actions to assess and improve population health and the well-being of the community. The next three provide a broad public health and systems context for impacting the social determinants of health. The three that follow focus on education and collaboration; one of these addresses health professional education in particular. The discussion then turns to two frameworks that expand upon educational concepts to include collaborations focused on interprofessional education and linkages among different sectors, respectively. Finally, two frameworks involve measuring aspects of health workforce development (health workers in underserved areas and social accountability of health professional schools) that are often overlooked in evaluations. All of these overarching categories are reflected in the committee's framework, which is presented in the next chapter.

PUTTING THE COMMUNITY IN CHARGE

The framework published by Audrey Danaher at the Wellesley Institute (see Figure 3-1) is part of a larger effort to reduce health disparities and improve population health through contributions from the community sector (Danaher, 2011). Within the context of the framework, the community sector is defined as "the wide range of not-for-profit organizations whose mandate is to work with and provide services to communities to meet local needs." As described in the box to the far right of the figure, a responsive and effective community sector can contribute to reducing health disparities. This is accomplished through direct community engagement that builds trust, provides services that ameliorate the impact of disparities, and mobilizes communities to influence policy on the social determinants of health as noted in the three center circles adjacent to the box. The far left circles describe the conditions in which the community sector functions: the top circle depicts the policies, economics, and social systems that give rise to

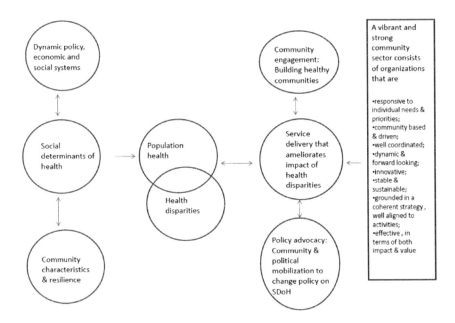

FIGURE 3-1 The Danaher framework.
NOTE: SDoH = social determinants of health.
SOURCE: Danaher, 2011. Reprinted with permission from the Wellesley Institute. For more information, visit http://www.wellesleyinstitute.com/wp-content/uploads/2011/10/Reducing-Disparities-and-Improving-Population-Health.pdf (accessed September 22, 2016).

the social determinants of health, and the bottom circle is the community characteristics that influence the social determinants of health.

As part of their guide to action on rural community health and well-being, researchers at Brandon University, the University of Manitoba, and Concordia University in Canada partnered with various stakeholder groups to build the framework seen in Figure 3-2 (Annis et al., 2004; Ryan-Nicholls, 2004). Stakeholders included

- rural community development corporations,
- regional health authorities,
- Community Futures Partners of Manitoba,

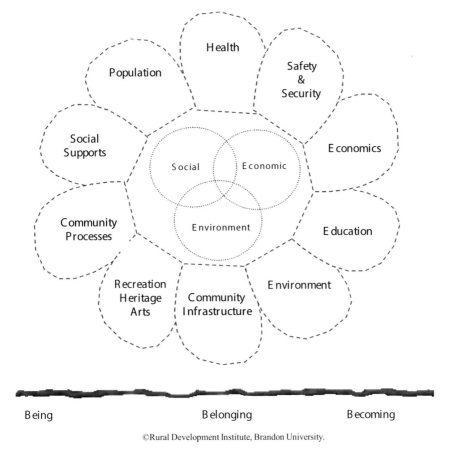

©Rural Development Institute, Brandon University.

FIGURE 3-2 Rural Community Health & Well-Being Framework.
SOURCE: Annis et al., 2004. Reprinted with permission from the Rural Development Institute and Brandon University.

- Wheat Belt Community Futures Development Corporation,
- Health Canada,
- the Rural Secretariat,
- Statistics Canada, and
- Brandon University researchers.

The purpose of the framework was to assist residents of rural communities in self-assessing quality-of-life measures that are listed under the framework as "Being," "Belonging," and "Becoming." *Being* involves understanding the current state of the community; *belonging* denotes how the community fits within the broader context; and *becoming* encompasses all the purposeful activities that are carried out to achieve the community's goals (Annis et al., 2004; Raphael et al., 1999).

In the center of the framework are the social, economic, and environmental factors that often predetermine a community's health and well-being. Stemming from these three circles are ten items that rural residents identified (and tested) as important considerations and additions to the framework. Each item is linked to an easily understood and interpreted indicator that has accessible and available data sources; measures what is important, credible, and acceptable to the residents of the rural community; and has a scientific, traditional, or community basis for inclusion that is considered reliable, trustworthy, and relevant. Through such an analysis of what is valued by rural communities, the residents themselves can begin to understand the current state of their community's health, well-being, and quality of life (Annis et al., 2004).

PUBLIC HEALTH AND SYSTEMS CONTEXT FOR IMPACTING THE SOCIAL DETERMINANTS OF HEALTH

In 2010, the World Health Organization (WHO) Commission on Social Determinants of Health published a conceptual framework for action on the social determinants of health (Solar and Irwin, 2010) that it used to orient its work, discussed in Chapter 1 (WHO, 2008). This framework is displayed in Figure 3-3 and is divided into structural and intermediary determinants. The structural determinants comprise the societal, economic, and political context in which a person is born and lives, which dictates one's socioeconomic position. One's socioeconomic position then sets the stage for the intermediary determinants (material circumstances, psychosocial circumstances, behavioral and/or biological factors, and the health system itself) and the likelihood of exposure to health-compromising conditions. Illnesses caused by poor living conditions can then circle back to the structural determinants if, for example, a person experiences a loss of employment or income, thereby lowering his or her socioeconomic status.

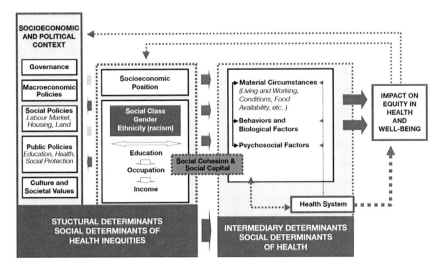

FIGURE 3-3 World Health Organization (WHO) conceptual framework.
SOURCE: Solar and Irwin, 2010. Reprinted with permission from the World Health
Organization.

Bridging the structural and intermediary determinants are concepts of social cohesion and social capital. The commissioners who developed the framework acknowledged that the inclusion of these concepts risked depoliticizing approaches to public health and the social determinants of health. However, they opted to include this bridge because they also believed that states could be in a position to promote equity through cooperative relationships between citizens and institutions by developing systems that would facilitate such connections. The final box to the far right of the figure shows the impacts of structural and intermediary determinants on equity in health and well-being and how those impacts can feed back to the structural determinants, having a positive, negative, or neutral influence on future generations.

Frieden (2010) developed a five-tier pyramid as a framework for improving public health (see Figure 3-4). Anchoring the base of the pyramid are interventions that Frieden states have the greatest potential impact on social determinants of health (e.g., poverty reduction, improved education). Next are interventions that benefit the vast majority of populations and are not labor-intensive, such as fluoridated water, followed by interventions that benefit large segments of the population and are more labor-intensive, such as immunizations. The tier above is direct clinical interventions for prevention of certain conditions, such as cardiovascular disease, that have

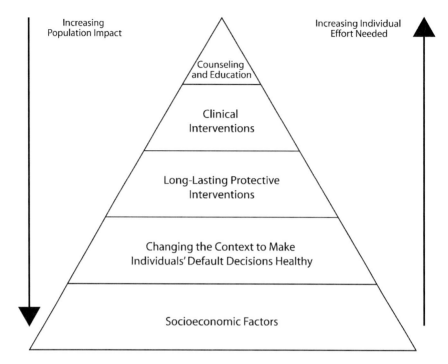

FIGURE 3-4 The Frieden framework.
SOURCE: Frieden, 2010. Reprinted with permission from the *American Journal of Public Health*.

the greatest health impact on individuals. Finally, at the top of the pyramid is education about health, which is believed to be the most labor-intensive intervention with the lowest public health impact.

According to Frieden (2010), since 1994, researchers have put forth public health frameworks that are similar but place greater emphasis on impacting health through clinical health services and the delivery of health care. Unlike these frameworks, Frieden used the social determinants of health to underpin his model.

Bay Area Regional Health Inequities Initiative is a group of local health departments in the San Francisco Bay Area dedicated to addressing health inequities. The initiative developed a health equity framework that depicts the link between health and social inequalities (see Figure 3-5). This framework shows upstream and downstream influences on health, as well as entry points for public health intervention. It broadens the scope of public health to include upstream drivers of health such as social inequities, institutional power, and living conditions (including physical, social,

59

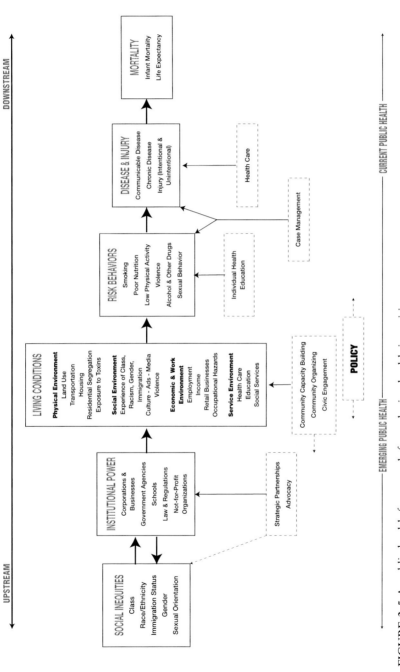

FIGURE 3-5 A public health framework for reducing health inequities.
SOURCE: BARHII, 2015. Reprinted with permission from the Bay Area Regional Health Inequities Initiative.

economic and work, and service environments). This framework has been formally adopted by the California Department of Public Health for application to its decision-making process (BARHII, 2015).

HEALTH PROFESSIONAL EDUCATION AND COLLABORATION

Karen Yoder (2006) developed a framework for service learning in dental education that could be applied to all health professions. Its focus is on planning, implementing, and evaluating service learning. It also allows educators to differentiate between service learning and other forms of

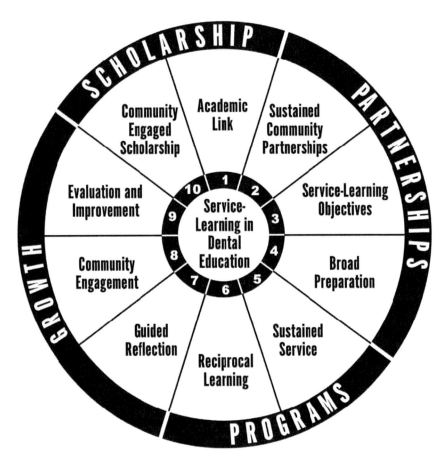

FIGURE 3-6 The Yoder framework.
SOURCE: Yoder, 2006. Reprinted with permission from the *Journal of Dental Education*.

community engagement, such as volunteerism, community service, internships, and field education, that may or may not include all the elements of true service learning (Furco, 1996). True service learning entails an ongoing synergistic effect between learning and service that involves active participation in thoughtfully organized service experiences deigned to meet the actual needs of the community. It also includes structured time for reflection and integration of the service into basic science and clinical courses (Chokshi, 2010; O'Brien et al., 2014; Yoder, 2006). The goal of service learning is to better prepare health professionals to work and partner effectively with diverse populations and communities, and to equip learners with competencies for interacting with other sectors, particularly within health policy.

As seen in Figure 3-6, service learning is placed in the center of the framework to signify an equal balance between service and learning and between the learner and the recipient of the service. The framework is structured around the four categories of scholarship, partnership, programs, and growth, each of which is further divided into two or three different but complementary components. In total, the framework encompasses ten essential components that are explained in Box 3-1.

Interprofessional education is key for helping health professionals learn to work with other professions and sectors. A previous Institute of Medicine (IOM) committee—the Committee on Measuring the Impact of Interprofessional Education on Collaborative Practice and Patient Outcomes—developed a model of interprofessional education (see Figure 3-7). This model depicts interprofessional education as ongoing and developing over time during a health professional's career, including both formal and informal education, as well as all stages of professional development (foundational education, graduate education, and continuing professional development). It includes four interrelated components: a learning continuum; the outcomes of learning; individual and population health outcomes; system outcomes such as organizational changes, system efficiencies, and cost-effectiveness; and the major enabling and interfering factors that influence implementation and overall outcomes (IOM, 2015, p. 28).

The Cooperative Extension (the Extension) developed a National Framework for Health and Wellness (see Figure 3-8) that is based on the National Prevention Council Action Plan of the U.S. Department of Health and Human Services (HHS, 2012). The HHS strategy identifies four areas for prevention efforts: (1) healthy and safe community environments, (2) clinical and community preventive services, (3) empowered people, and (4) elimination of health disparities (HHS, 2012). These areas are captured in the center of the Extension's framework, in the overall goal to "increase the number of Americans who are healthy at every stage of life" (ECOP Task Force, 2014).

BOX 3-1
10 Components of Service Learning

Scholarship
1. Academic link: "Service combined with learning adds value to each and transforms both" (p. 116).
2. Community-engaged scholarship: "A significant gap exists between the goal of health professional schools to function as community-engaged institutions and the reality of how faculty members are typically judged and rewarded, which often does not value service to the community" (p. 121).

Partnerships
3. Sustained community partnerships: "The assignments may be consistent with the service-learning method, in which emphasis is placed on developing a few, high-quality, equal, ongoing relationships with selected community partners" (p. 117).
4. Service learning objectives: "Faculty and community partners should jointly formulate learning and service objectives to describe what service they will be providing and how this experience connects with their learning" (p. 118).
5. Broad preparation: "Broad preparation provides students with information that will help them understand the form and function of the agency or institution they will service and the people with whom they will interact" (p. 119).

Programs
6. Sustained service: "Unlike assignments to provide an educational presentation in a classroom, service-learning involves a sustained amount of time in preparation and service" (p. 119).
7. Reciprocal learning: "Alert students to the expectation of learning from the community partner mentors who are highly skilled in working with special populations" (p. 119).

Growth
8. Guided reflection: "Guided reflection causes students to make the connection between their service and academic objectives and fosters the exploration and clarification of complex social issues and personal values" (p. 119).
9. Community engagement: "Community engagement is meant to include knowledge about the cultural components of the community and involvement in advocating for health policy issues that affect that community" (p. 120).
10. Evaluation and improvement: "Because service-learning programs often involve external funding, the evaluation process can be an effective tool for demonstrating outcomes of the program and encouraging continued funding" (p. 121).

SOURCE: Excerpted from Yoder, 2006.

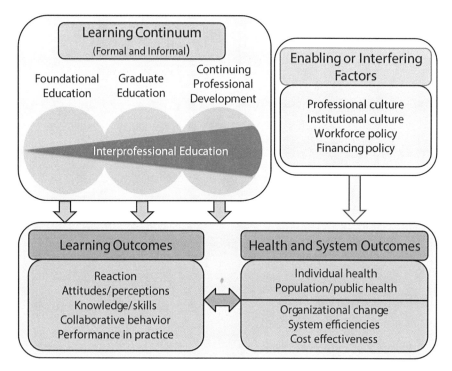

FIGURE 3-7 The interprofessional learning continuum model.
NOTE: For this model, "graduate education" encompasses any advanced formal or supervised health professional training taking place between the completion of foundational education and entry into unsupervised practice.
SOURCE: IOM, 2015.

The Extension's framework also is based on the social-ecological model of Urie Bronfenbrenner (1979), which addresses the relationships among individual, community, and societal factors. That model is captured in the first ring of the framework, "healthy and safe environments" and "healthy and safe choices." The next ring depicts the Extension's six priority areas: health policy issues education; integrated nutrition, health, environment, and agriculture systems; health literacy; chronic disease prevention and management; positive youth development for health; and health insurance literacy. The outer ring identifies key partners with which to collaborate to achieve the Extension's goals: an engaged university system, health professionals, the education sector, the private sector, the public sector, engaged communities, community organizations, and clinical and community preventive services (ECOP Task Force, 2014).

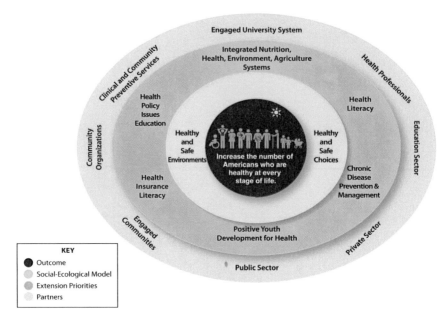

FIGURE 3-8 The Cooperative Extension's National Framework for Health and Wellness.
SOURCE: ECOP Task Force, 2014. Reprinted with permission from the Extension Committee on Organization and Policy Health Task Force. For more information, visit http://www.aplu.org/members/commissions/food-environment-and-renewable-resources/CFERR_Library/national-framework-for-health-and-wellness/file (accessed September 22, 2016).

MONITORING AND EVALUATION

Figure 3-9 depicts a conceptual framework for measuring efforts to increase access to health workers in underserved areas. This framework builds on previous monitoring and evaluation efforts of WHO (2009) and parallels the WHO Commission's social, political, and economic context as illustrated in Figure 3-3. These contextual factors are rarely considered in evaluations of country-led initiatives to attract and retain qualified health workers in underserved areas. Huicho and colleagues (2010) proposed this framework to capture contextual factors and overcome evaluation challenges due to the complexity of interventions and the lack of previously published guidelines.

Based on a systems approach, this framework is divided into inputs (design and implementation), outputs, outcomes, and impact. For each of

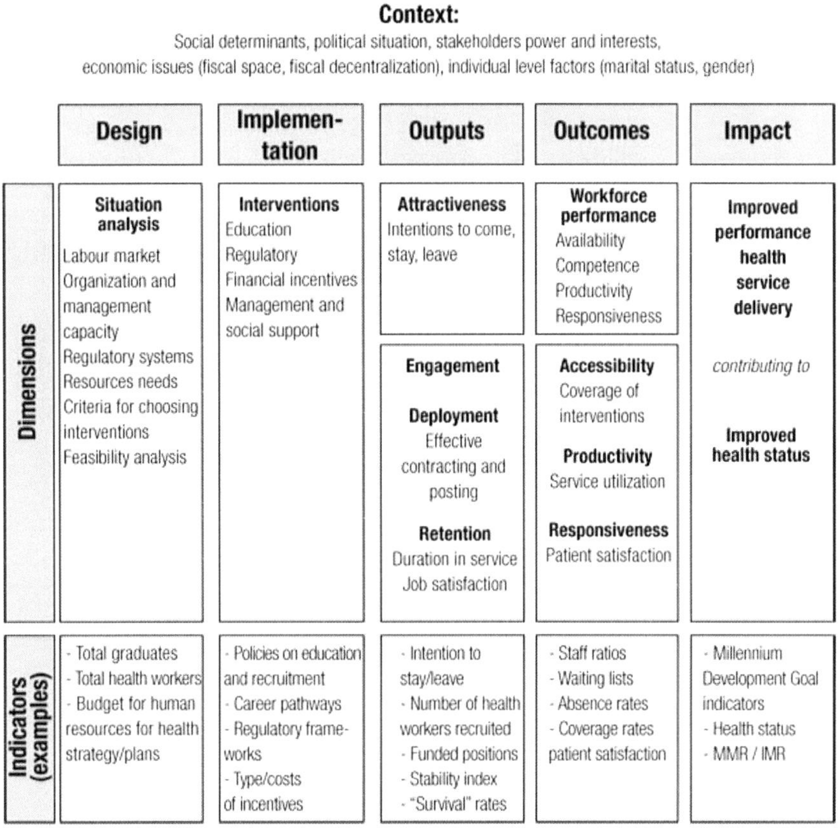

Context:
Social determinants, political situation, stakeholders power and interests,
economic issues (fiscal space, fiscal decentralization), individual level factors (marital status, gender)

	Design	Implemen-tation	Outputs	Outcomes	Impact
Dimensions	**Situation analysis** Labour market Organization and management capacity Regulatory systems Resources needs Criteria for choosing interventions Feasibility analysis	**Interventions** Education Regulatory Financial incentives Management and social support	**Attractiveness** Intentions to come, stay, leave **Engagement** **Deployment** Effective contracting and posting **Retention** Duration in service Job satisfaction	**Workforce performance** Availability Competence Productivity Responsiveness **Accessibility** Coverage of interventions **Productivity** Service utilization **Responsiveness** Patient satisfaction	**Improved performance health service delivery** *contributing to* **Improved health status**
Indicators (examples)	- Total graduates - Total health workers - Budget for human resources for health strategy/plans	- Policies on education and recruitment - Career pathways - Regulatory frame-works - Type/costs of incentives	- Intention to stay/leave - Number of health workers recruited - Funded positions - Stability index - "Survival" rates	- Staff ratios - Waiting lists - Absence rates - Coverage rates patient satisfaction	- Millennium Development Goal indicators - Health status - MMR / IMR

FIGURE 3-9 A conceptual framework for measuring efforts to increase access to health workers in underserved areas.
NOTE: IMR = infant mortality rate; MMR = maternal mortality ratio.
SOURCE: Huicho et al., 2010. Reprinted with permission from the World Health Organization.

these divisions, the authors provide examples of indicators for evaluating success. Of particular interest for purposes of this report is the emphasis on education during the input phase, retention of workers as an output, worker performance as an outcome, and improved health status as a measurable impact (Huicho et al., 2010).

Finally, THEnet created a comprehensive framework to aid schools in examining and learning how to improve health outcomes and health systems performance. This framework is designed to be useful at the individual school level, the network/partnership level, and the broader level. Its

---

BOX 3-2
The Social Accountability Framework for
Health Workforce Training

Section 1: What needs are we addressing? This section asks schools to consider their role in addressing the health and social needs of the reference population, the health workforce needs, and the health system needs. It asks the school to define the communities they serve, identify the priority health and social needs, as well as the needs of the health system.

Section 2: How do we work? This section addresses important aspects of the organization and planning, and asks schools to assess their values, governance, and decision-making processes and their partnerships with the health sector, community groups, and policy makers.

Section 3: What do we do? This section focuses on the school's program including composition of students and teachers, curriculum, learning methodologies, research, service, and resource allocation.

Section 4: What difference do we make? This section asks schools to consider their graduates, where they are, and their practice. Plus, to consider engagement with and impact on health services and community, their cost effectiveness, and their influence in assisting other schools toward becoming more socially accountable.

SOURCE: Excerpted from THEnet, 2015.

---

purpose is to help schools assess their social accountability, and it is structured around a series of questions under four sections, presented in Box 3-2 (THEnet, 2015). The entire framework is accessible online (THEnet, 2015).

REFERENCES

Annis, R., F. Racher, and M. Beattie. 2004. *Rural community health and well-being: A guide to action*. Brandon, Manitoba: Rural Development Institute. https://www.brandonu.ca/rdi/publication/rural-community-health-and-well-being-a-guide-to-action (accessed September 22, 2016).

BARHII (Bay Area Regional Health Inequities Initiative). 2015. *A public health framework for reducing health inequities*. http://barhii.org/framework (accessed September 22, 2016).

Bronfenbrenner, U. 1979. *The ecology of human development*. Cambridge, MA: Harvard University Press.

Chokshi, D. A. 2010. Teaching about health disparities using a social determinants framework. *Journal of General Internal Medicine* 25(Suppl. 2):S182-S185.

Danaher, A. 2011. *Reducing disparities and improving population health: The role of a vibrant community sector.* Toronto, ON: Wellesley Institute. http://www.wellesleyinstitute.com/wp-content/uploads/2011/10/Reducing-Disparities-and-Improving-Population-Health.pdf (accessed September 22, 2016).

ECOP (Extension Committee on Organization and Policy) Task Force. 2014. *Cooperative Extension's national framework for health and wellness.* http://www.aplu.org/members/commissions/food-environment-and-renewable-resources/CFERR_Library/national-framework-for-health-and-wellness/file (accessed December 9, 2015).

Frieden, T. R. 2010. A framework for public health action: The health impact pyramid. *American Journal of Public Health* 100(4):590-595.

Furco, A. 1996. Service-learning: A balanced approach to experiential education. In *Expanding boundaries: Serving and learning*, edited by B. Taylor. Washington, DC: Corporation for National Service. Pp. 2-6.

HHS (U.S. Department of Health and Human Services). 2012. *National Prevention Council Action Plan: Implementing the national prevention strategy.* Washington, DC: HHS.

Huicho, L., M. Dieleman, J. Campbell, L. Codjia, D. Balabanova, G. Dussault, and C. Dolea. 2010. Increasing access to health workers in underserved areas: A conceptual framework for measuring results. *Bulletin of the World Health Organization* 88(5):357-363.

IOM (Institute of Medicine). 2015. *Measuring the impact of interprofessional education on collaborative practice and patient outcomes.* Washington, DC: The National Academies Press.

O'Brien, M. J., J. M. Garland, K. M. Murphy, S. J. Shuman, R. C. Whitaker, and S. C. Larson. 2014. Training medical students in the social determinants of health: The Health Scholars Program at Puentes de Salud. *Advances in Medical Education and Practice* 5:307-314.

Raphael, D., I. Brown, and R. Renwick. 1999. Psychometric properties of the full and short versions of the quality of life instrument package: Results from the Ontario Province-Wide Study. *International Journal of Disability, Development and Education* 46(2):157-168.

Ryan-Nicholls, K. 2004. Rural Canadian community health and quality of life: Testing a workbook to determine priorities and move to action. *Rural Remote Health* 4(2):278.

Solar, O., and A. Irwin. 2010. *A conceptual framework for action on the social determinants of health. Social determinants of health discussion paper 2 (policy and practice).* Geneva, Switzerland: WHO. http://www.who.int/sdhconference/resources/ConceptualframeworkforactiononSDH_eng.pdf (accessed September 22, 2016).

THEnet (The Training for Health Equity Network). 2015. *The social accountability framework for health workforce training.* http://thenetcommunity.org/social-accountability-framework (accessed January 7, 2016).

WHO (World Health Organization). 2008. *Closing the gap in a generation: Health equity through action on the social determinants of health, final report.* Geneva, Switzerland: WHO Commission on Social Determinants of Health.

WHO. 2009. *Monitoring and Evaluation Working Group of the International Health Partnership and related initiatives (IHP+). Monitoring performance and evaluating progress in the scale-up for better health: A proposed common framework.* Geneva, Switzerland: WHO.

Yoder, K. M. 2006. A framework for service-learning in dental education. *Journal of Dental Education* 70(2):115-123.

4

Social Determinants of Health: A Framework for Educating Health Professionals

SUMMARY

The previous two chapters explore how the education of health professionals is currently addressing the social determinants of health in and with communities. What becomes apparent is that education in the social determinants of health is not part of a broader, systematic approach. Rather, there is a need for a holistic, consistent, coherent structure aligning education, health, and other sectors in partnership with communities. To help meet this need, the committee developed a framework for strengthening the education of health professionals to impart better understanding the social determinants of health across the learning continuum. This framework comprises three domains (education, community, and organization), collectively encompassing nine components. Three key concepts—transformative learning, dynamic partnerships, and lifelong learning—underpin the framework and appear, both explicitly and implicitly, throughout the descriptions of the three domains. Further, because the framework is only a small fraction of the universe of requirements for a sustainable impact on the social determinants of health, the committee also created a model depicting how the framework fits within the broader social, political, and economic contexts. This model draws on the World Health Organization's conceptual framework, described in Chapter 3. Linked to the framework and the model are four recommendations directed at a wide array of actors, with a focus on those groups identified in Chapter 1 (e.g., signatories of the Rio Declaration and the sponsors of this study) that are calling for education and action on the social determinants of health.

A UNIFYING FRAMEWORK

Based on its review of the literature and multiple calls for action, the committee concludes that there is a need and a demand for a holistic, consistent, coherent structure that aligns education, health, and other sectors to better meet local needs in partnership with communities. This conclusion informed the committee's vision for inspiring health professionals to engage in action on the social determinants of health while providing an educational structure for understanding a systems-based approach for such action.

Elements of a Unifying Framework

Chapter 3 presents a number of prior frameworks salient to understanding and acting on the social determinants of health. Each has particular strengths that, when combined, fulfill the committee's vision for better aligning different sectors in educating health professionals to address the social determinants of health in partnership with communities. Overlaying this vision are Frenk and colleagues' (2010) proposed instructional and institutional reforms for achieving "transformative and interdependent professional education for equity in health" (p. 1953). The actions taken to produce enlightened change agents who are innovative, adaptive, and responsive to the needs of the community is what these authors identify as "transformative learning."[1] Transformative learning, dynamic partnerships, and lifelong learning are fundamental principles underpinning the committee's framework.

Transformative Learning

Transformative learning is key to addressing the social determinants of health. It involves vital shifts that would move health professional education from a traditional biomedical-centric approach to an approach that can provide a greater understanding of and competencies in addressing complex health systems in an increasingly global and interconnected world. Building upon the work of the *Lancet* Commission (Frenk et al., 2010), described in Chapter 1, the committee proposes a list of desired education outcomes from transformative learning that include competency to

- search, analyze, and synthesize information for decision making;
- collaborate and partner effectively with others;

---

[1] For the purposes of this report, the terms "transformative learning" and "transformative education" are considered interchangeable.

- work with, understand, and value the vital role of all players within health systems and other sectors that impact health; and
- apply global efforts addressing health inequities to local priorities and actions.

Dynamic Partnerships

Dynamic partnerships also are key to effectively addressing the social determinants of health. These partnerships entail close working relationships among policy makers, educators, health professionals, community organizations, nonhealth professionals, and community members. Health professionals who are educated under what Frenk and colleagues (2010) term the "traditional model" of education—which focuses more on what is taught and by whom rather than on building relevant competencies— are unlikely to experience the exposure to the broader social, political, and environmental contexts provided by education from a wide array of partners. And innovative methods of education challenge learners to solve problems and make new connections through exposure to other professions, sectors, and populations. The bidirectional linkages formed between communities and educators reinforce equality in the partnership, which can be strengthened through mutual support among communities, educators, and organizations (Tan et al., 2013).

Lifelong Learning

The European Council Resolution on Lifelong Learning (Council of the European Union, 2002) describes lifelong learning as a continuum of learning throughout the life course aimed at "improving knowledge, skills and competences within a personal, civic, social and/or employment-related perspective" (p. C163/2). It involves formal education as well as nonformal and informal learning opportunities, as defined in a 2015 United Nations Educational, Scientific and Cultural Organization (UNESCO) report (Yang, 2015). That report describes how lifelong learning, through the development and recognition of learners' knowledge, skills, and competences, is gaining relevance for poverty reduction, job creation, employment, and social inclusion, all of which represent potential impacts on the social determinants of health.

As part of lifelong learning, nonformal education and informal learning opportunities create space for university–community partnerships to address the social determinants of health. Men's Sheds, for example, are community-based organizations that began in Australia and have expanded around the world to offer older men a place to use, develop, and share such skills as furniture making (Wilson and Cordier, 2013). Health and social policy makers use these venues to engage men and promote health and well-being outside of traditional health and care settings (Wilson and Cordier, 2013). Wilson and Cordier propose incorporating the social determinants of health and well-being in study designs to better analyze the health impacts of informal learning in Men's Sheds. For the health professions, continuing professional development/continuing education and problem-based learning are often regarded as approaches to lifelong learning (FIP, 2014; Josiah Macy Jr. Foundation, 2010; Lane, 2008; Wood, 2003).

Domains of the Framework

Combining transformative learning, dynamic partnerships, and lifelong learning with key aspects of the frameworks presented in Chapter 3 (i.e., putting the community in charge, public health and systems context, health professional education and collaboration, and monitoring and evaluation), the committee developed a unifying framework for educating health professionals to address the social determinants of health (see Figure 4-1). For the

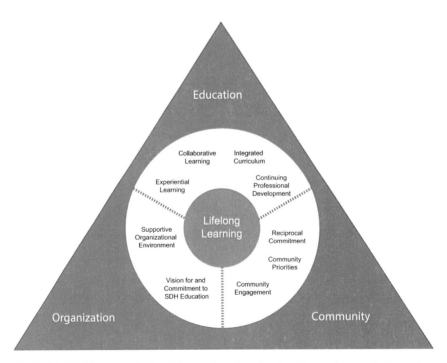

FIGURE 4-1 Framework for lifelong learning for health professionals in understanding and addressing the social determinants of health.
NOTE: SDH = social determinants of health.

impact of this framework to be fully realized, health professionals will need access to education that builds critical thinking through transformative learning opportunities, from foundational education through continuing professional development. Such education is built around three domains:

1. education
2. community
3. organization

EDUCATION

The sorts of activities the committee believes serve as elements of transformative learning for addressing the social determinants of health go well beyond traditional lecturing. The committee views an approach to such transformative learning as involving creating, through education, highly competent professionals who understand and act on the social determinants of health in ways that advance communities and individuals toward greater health equity. Box 4-1 lists components of that education, which are discussed below.

BOX 4-1
Components of the Education Domain

Experiential learning
  • Applied learning
  • Community engagement
  • Performance assessment

Collaborative learning
  • Problem/project-based learning
  • Student engagement
  • Critical thinking

Integrated curriculum
  • Interprofessional
  • Cross-sectoral
  • Longitudinally organized

Continuing professional development
  • Faculty development
  • Interprofessional workplace learning

Experiential Learning

Experiential learning is a vital component of education in how to apply understanding of the social determinants of health (Cené et al., 2010; McIntosh et al., 2008; McNeil et al., 2013). In 1984, Robert Kolb designed the Experiential Learning Cycle, which emphasizes that such education is effective only if learners are fully and openly involved in new experiences without bias and are provided time to reflect upon and observe their experience from many perspectives (Kolb, 1984). It is through experiential opportunities, combined with reflection, that learners develop and strengthen their competency for self-examination of personally held assumptions, values, and beliefs about individuals and populations. Exploration of one's biases and positions needs to continue throughout life, reaching deeper levels as the health professional matures cognitively, personally, and professionally (El-Sayed and El-Sayed, 2014). Faculty and other educators similarly need to reflect upon their personal views, particularly with respect to the changing student population, which in some cases includes young people whose learning styles differ from those of prior generations and in other cases includes both more mature learners who bring substantial previous work experience and more entrants from overseas (Newman and Peile, 2002; Regan-Smith, 1998).

Applied Learning

Applied learning is a particular form of experiential learning that puts principles into practice through a mixed-methods pedagogical approach. It has a strong educational component that distinguishes it from volunteerism (Schwartzman and Henry, 2009). Given the lack of oversight and accountability in volunteer activities, the value to the community of purely altruistic activities by students and culturally unaware health professionals is suspect, and such activities may even be counterproductive (Caldron et al., 2015). An example of applied learning is service learning that places equal emphasis on service and on learning for the benefit of all parties involved (Furco, 1996).

Community Engagement

Strasser and colleagues (2015) explore relationships between communities and medical education programs. Such relationships have evolved from community-oriented activities in the 1960s and 1970s, to community-based interventions in the 1980s and 1990s, to the twenty-first-century concept of community-engaged education. Community engagement denotes service learning activities that stress reciprocity and interdependence in mutually beneficial partnerships between academic institutions and the communities in which they reside (Furco, 1996; Sigmon, 1979).

Performance Assessment

Performance assessment of the competency of health professionals, students, and trainees in addressing the social determinants of health entails demonstrating competencies articulated for transformative learning. The expectations for such competencies in performance assessment deepen in complexity as learners mature and progress from foundational education to continuing professional development, and as their experiences with the social determinants of health broaden. The 360-degree multisource feedback model is one method used to garner a wide array of inputs for assessment of professionalism and teaching, as well as for program evaluation (Berk, 2009; Donnon et al., 2014; Richmond et al., 2011).

Collaborative Learning

There are a variety of approaches to collaborative learning (Dillenbourg, 1999). The unifying factor for all of these approaches is an emphasis on group work that involves students co-learning with each other, communities, and health professionals who also learn from each other (Dooly, 2008). In the field of public health, in which learners grow to understand how to address problems within complex systems, learning how to work collaboratively with other professions and other sectors is critical (Carman, 2015; Kickbusch, 2013; Levy et al., 2015; Lomazzi et al., 2016). But all health professionals are increasingly being called upon to work collaboratively with other professions. Engaging students through interprofessional projects in and with communities can help build the capacity of the health workforce for understanding and acting on the social determinants of health.

Problem/Project-Based Learning and Critical Thinking

Problem-based learning is generally viewed by students as beneficial and can promote a desire to learn (Barman et al., 2006; Cónsul-Giribet and Medina-Moya, 2014). Such learning provides opportunities to build competencies in communication, problem solving, teamwork, and collaboration involving mutual respect for others (Wood, 2003). With this pedagogy, learners develop critical thinking skills through learner-centered approaches that reflect real world situations (Ivicek et al., 2011; Shreeve, 2008).

Problem/Project-Based Learning and Student Engagement

At McMaster University, where problem-based learning originated, students are presented with individually designed problems to stimulate and guide their learning. Each problem varies with regard to group sizes and the incorporation of other pedagogy, but each follows a similar process that requires active student engagement through self-study and guidance by educators who establish clear learning objectives for the activity (Walsh, 2005). Problem-based learning has shown positive impacts on critical thinking and movement toward lifelong learning; given the self-directed nature of the activity, however, obtaining its full benefit requires diligence in maintaining the processes involved (Khoiriyah et al., 2015).

Project-based learning is an adaptation of problem-based learning whereby students are challenged to confront real situations so as to acquire a deeper understanding of such situations (Edutopia, 2016; Thomas, 2000). As such, project-based learning can be considered a useful tool for educating health professionals in addressing the social determinants of health in and with communities.

Integrated Curriculum

Multiple perspectives on what constitutes an integrated curriculum have led to varying definitions of the term (Brauer and Ferguson, 2015; Howard et al., 2009; Pearson and Hubball, 2012). Broadening Brauer and Ferguson's (2015) proposed definition of the term for medical education, the committee considers it to mean an interprofessional approach for delivery of information and experiences that combines basic and applied concepts throughout all years of foundational education.

Interprofessional and Cross-Sectoral[2] Curriculum

The development of competencies to engage interprofessionally and across sectors in partnership with communities and community organizations is an important element of transformative learning for addressing the social determinants of health. Providing interprofessional opportunities presents logistical and social challenges (Anderson et al., 2010; Cashman et al., 2004) that are distinct from the challenges of community-engaged learning opportunities (Michener et al., 2012; Strasser et al., 2015). But as the service-learning home visitation program of Florida International

---

[2] The committee envisions a health workforce that is proactive in addressing and acting on the social determinants of health, and therefore elected to take a cross-sectoral approach rather than the intersectoral approach taken by the World Health Organization (WHO) and the *Lancet* Commission.

University and other such programs demonstrate, the potential gains that accrue from learning from and with other professions and other sectors can be powerful educational tools (Art et al., 2007; Bainbridge et al., 2014; Mihalynuk et al., 2007; Ross et al., 2014). In the case of the Florida International University program, medical, nursing, social work, and law students, plus faculty, work together in addressing patients' nonhealth needs so as to improve their health. This interprofessional and cross-sectoral outreach to individual community members has resulted in greater adherence to preventive health measures and a tendency to make fewer trips to the emergency room compared with individual households that received minimal intervention (Rock et al., 2014). Some entire programs have been designed around transdisciplinary problem solving in public health, while in other cases, the overall educational strategy has been reshaped to promote competencies across fields through transformative learning and integrated instructional design methods (Frenk et al., 2015; Lawlor et al., 2015).

Longitudinally Organized Curriculum

Creating a longitudinal curriculum for the social determinants of health conveys to students the importance of the topic for their professional development (Doran et al., 2008), and allows learning objectives to build and increase in complexity as students advance in their professional development and maturity. In a review of the literature using the BEME (Best Evidence Medical and Health Professional Education) review guidelines, Thistlethwaite and colleagues (2013) found that for most medical students, longitudinal placements (including both community and hospital placements) varied in length from one half-day per week for 6 months to full-time immersion for more than 12 months. The University of Michigan Medical School organizes a required Poverty in Healthcare curriculum that runs throughout the 4 years of education (Doran et al., 2008).

Continuing Professional Development

Faculty Development

Faculty development is one way in which leadership and organizations can demonstrate their support for educators wishing to offer interprofessional, community-engaged learning. Possessing the skills to offer transformative learning opportunities is essential not only for university faculty but also for community volunteers and preceptors, who are often geographically dispersed, diverse in their backgrounds and experience, and challenged by intense time and resource pressures (Langlois and Thach, 2003). Langlois and Thach suggest practical strategies for overcoming some of these barriers, such as offering "just in time" training, providing a variety of educational formats, and linking training to continuing education credits.

Toolkits for quality improvement of education in community facilities (Malik et al., 2007), workplace learning, and learning communities may offer additional strategies for skill and knowledge acquisition by university and community-based faculty and volunteers (Chou et al., 2014; Lloyd et al., 2014; O'Sullivan and Irby, 2011). On-site training that allows workers at understaffed organizations to remain at the workplace for training is a viable option, particularly for low-resource settings (Burnett et al., 2015).

Interprofessional Workplace Learning

According to Lloyd and colleagues (2014), learning in the workplace can be formal, as in the case of an invited speaker, or informal, as when peers come together spontaneously to reflect upon an incident. While some have proposed informal workplace learning as a method for interprofessional education, it remains a relatively untapped opportunity for sharing learning across professions (Kitto et al., 2014; Mulder et al., 2010; Nisbet et al., 2013). Making interprofessional workplace learning more integral to everyday practice is a way of supplying busy providers of health care and social support with real-time education and interactions with respect to how social, political, and economic conditions impact the health of individuals and populations. However, insufficient staffing and heavy workloads can impede even informal educational opportunities (Lloyd et al., 2014; Wahab et al., 2014). Leaders who are supported by their organizations can create space to encourage such interactions.

Recommendation

Introducing any of the components discussed above into health professional education would represent a move toward transformative learning, but for maximal impact, the committee makes the following recommendation:

Recommendation 1: Health professional educators should use the framework presented in this report as a guide for creating lifelong learners who appreciate the value of relationships and collaborations for understanding and addressing community-identified needs and for strengthening community assets.

Implementing the committee's framework would enable health professional students, trainees, educators, practitioners, researchers, and policy makers to understand the social determinants of health. It also would enable them to form appropriate partnerships for taking action on the social determinants of health by engaging in experiential learning that includes reflective observations; promoting collaborative, interprofessional, and cross-sectoral engagements for addressing the social determinants; and partnering with individuals and communities to address health inequities.

To demonstrate effective implementation of the framework, health professional educators should

- publish literature on analyses of and lessons learned from curricula that offer learning opportunities that are responsive to the evolving needs and assets of local communities; and
- document case studies of health professional advocacy using a health-in-all-policies approach.[3]

COMMUNITY

Partnerships with communities are an essential part of educating health professionals in the social determinants of health. The community becomes an equal partner in teaching health professionals, faculty, and students about its experiences and how the social determinants have shaped the lives of its members. In this way, community members educate health professionals about the priorities of the community in addressing disparities stemming from the social determinants of health. Through shifts in power from health professionals to community members and organizations, the community shares responsibility for developing strategies for the creation of learning opportunities that can advance health equity based on community priorities. Box 4-2 outlines the three identified domain components that are essential for partnerships with communities.

Reciprocal Commitment

To better understand the goals of service learning and community-based medical education, Hunt and colleagues (2011) conducted a systematic review of the literature. The authors report enthusiasm among educators for employing community-based education as a method for teaching the social determinants of health, but found little evidence that community members were routinely involved in identifying local health priorities. This situation is not unique to medicine. Taylor and Le Riche (2006) looked at the equality of partnerships between service users and carers in social work

---

[3] "Health in all policies" denotes an approach to policies or reforms that is designed to achieve healthier communities by integrating public health actions with primary care and by pursuing healthy public policies across sectors (WHO, 2008a, 2011a).

BOX 4-2
Components of the Community Domain

Reciprocal commitment
- Community assets
- Willingness to engage
- Networks
- Resources

Community priorities
- Evaluation of health impacts toward equity and well-being

Community engagement
- Workforce diversity
- Recruitment and retention

---

education. They suggest that effective strategies are needed for "improving the quality of partnerships working in education, and health and social care practice" (p. 418). However, they also point out that research in this area is lacking, which influenced their findings. One positive finding came from a study of service-learning activities at Morehouse School of Medicine aimed at addressing health disparities among underserved youth and adults (Buckner et al., 2010). These authors define success as the commitment from community organizations to engage in activities with students for multiple years. According to Strasser and colleagues (2015), such reciprocal commitment between communities and universities involves open and level communication with community leaders and members so that assumptions can be challenged in an effort to understand the perspectives of all stakeholders (Strasser et al., 2015).

While service-learning projects and community-based education serve as an effective bridge between the classroom and the community, such programs often train students in how to educate communities instead of empowering communities to educate current and future health professionals. Learning how to educate and learning how to listen are equally important for health professionals, students, and trainees if they are to work effectively in and with communities.

Community Assets

An often-cited study by McKnight and Kretzmann (1990) identifies the "deficiency-oriented social service model" as a source for thinking of low-income neighborhoods as needy rather than as resources for improving quality of life. The result is a *needs* assessment that identifies, quantifies, and maps problems faced by a community, such as a high crime rate, low literacy, and poor health outcomes. In contrast, mapping even the poorest community's assets, capacities, and abilities places within the community the locus of control for building upon existing resources and incorporating new ones. Neighborhood asset mapping is used around the world for actively engaging communities on such topics as obesity (Economos and Irish-Hauser, 2007), diabetes (Kelley et al., 2005), mental health (Selamu et al., 2015), and chronic disease prevention (Santilli et al., 2011). For its chronic disease prevention activity, for example, the Yale School of Public Health employed local high school students to conduct asset mapping. By partnering with youth leadership development organizations, the Yale researchers gained valuable information about community assets while employing youth and gaining entry into what Santilli and colleagues (2011) describe as "some of New Haven's most research-wary and skeptical neighborhoods" (p. 2209).

In 2005, the W.K. Kellogg Foundation supported development of the Asset-Based Community Development (ABCD) Institute's guide to mobilizing local assets and organizational capacity (Kretzmann et al., 2005). This guide identifies five categories of community assets (see Box 4-3). These categories can guide universities in characterizing community assets in order to strengthen stakeholder partnerships through community engagement.

Willingness to Engage

Community mistrust of academic institutions is an impediment to forming sustainable academic–community partnerships for addressing the social determinants of health that lead to health disparities (Abdulrahim et al., 2010; Christopher et al., 2008; Goldberg-Freeman et al., 2007; Jagosh et al., 2015). Given the history of exploitative research in disadvantaged communities, such mistrust is understandable, but it also impedes valuable research that could eliminate health disparities (Christopher et al., 2008).

Community-based participatory research is an approach to designing studies that builds and maintains community trust through equitable involvement of all partners in the research process (NIH OBSSR, n.d.). With this approach, community members and researchers work together to construct, analyze, interpret, and communicate the study findings. The combination of shared knowledge and a desire for action is the engine for social change that improves community health and reduces health disparities. Numerous groups around the world have used community-based participatory research to build community trust in research aimed at improving health, equity, and quality of life in communities (Abdulrahim et

---

BOX 4-3
Five Categories of Community Assets

1. Local residents—their skills, experiences, passions, capacities and willing-ness to contribute to the project. Special attention is paid to residents who are sometimes "marginalized."

2. Local voluntary associations, clubs, and networks—e.g., all of the athletic, cul-tural, social, faith-based, etc., groups powered by volunteer members—which might contribute to the project.

3. Local institutions—e.g., public institutions such as schools, libraries, parks, police stations, etc., along with local businesses and non-profits—which might contribute to the project.

4. Physical assets—e.g., the land, the buildings, the infrastructure, transportation, etc., which might contribute to the project.

5. Economic assets—e.g., what people produce and consume, businesses, in-formal economic exchanges, barter relationships, etc.

SOURCE: Excerpted from Kretzmann et al., 2005, pp. 1-2.

---

al., 2010; Metzler et al., 2003; Mosavel et al., 2005; Teufel-Shone et al., 2006; Wallerstein and Duran, 2010).

Networks and Resources

Formal and informal networks provide resources for meeting the daily needs of communities (McLeroy et al., 2003). During the HIV epidemic in sub-Saharan Africa, for example, the church was frequently identified as a formal pathway to HIV prevention, treatment, and impact mitigation (Campbell et al., 2013a,b; Murray et al., 2011). Other formal networks include schools, businesses, voluntary agencies, and political structures. Within formal structures are informal social networks formed among fami-lies, neighborhoods, and populations that share unique characteristics. These informal support systems hold potential solutions to better meeting the needs of community members. However, researchers' access to these less formal networks require an insider's understanding of the commu-nity (McLeroy et al., 2003). Funneling resources through informal net-works arguably strengthens researchers' access to and collaborations with communities.

Community Priorities

Community-based research differs from community-based participatory research. The former indicates only the locus of the activity, whereas the latter empowers communities to engage fully with the research being undertaken in their community (Blumenthal, 2011). While community-based participatory research is an ethical approach that empowers communities, it does present some risk to the researcher when community priorities do not match those of the researcher or even involve health (Williams et al., 2009). Balancing community priorities with the interests and skill set of the academic researcher requires careful negotiation among all parties, including the organizations funding and supporting the work (Rhodes et al., 2010).

One way to ensure that research reflects community priorities while further enhancing the education of health professionals in the social determinants of health is by conducting health impact assessments (HIAs)—in depth examinations of policies, programs, or projects for their effects on population health (Bhatia et al., 2014; WHO European Centre for Health Policy, 1999). HIAs have been used worldwide within the context of a health-in-all-policies approach to explore potential unintended consequences of policies and initiatives for the health of populations or segments thereof (Collins and Koplan, 2009; Leppo et al., 2013). This cross-sector approach has been adopted by groups throughout the world to improve population health and health equity. With this approach, public policies are analyzed systematically for their potential effects on health determinants. The findings of such analyses can be used to hold policy makers accountable for the health impacts of policies they promote (Leppo et al., 2013). The University of Wisconsin Department of Population Health Sciences incorporated both service learning and HIAs in its master's-level public health course to generate knowledge, as well as to build a foundation for community partnerships (Feder et al., 2013).

According to Heller and colleagues (2014), "the process of conducting an HIA can build or strengthen relationships between stakeholders and can engage and empower populations who are likely to be affected by a proposal and who may already face poor health outcomes and marginalization. HIAs often recognize the lived experience of those populations as important evidence" (p. 11054). The authors propose incorporating equity considerations into HIA practice so that impacts of policy and planning decisions on population subgroups can be traced and then used to empower marginalized communities so as to promote and protect health equity (Heller et al., 2014). To measure progress toward this goal, the authors developed equity metrics that comprise "a measurement scale, examples of high scoring activities, potential data sources, and example interview questions to gather data and guide evaluators on scoring each metric" (Heller et al., 2014, p. 11055). The health professions might consider these metrics for use in guiding the development of desired competencies for partnering with communities to address the social determinants of health.

Community Engagement

Increasing the representation of indigenous and minority populations in health professional education and practice is critical to addressing the social determinants of health that lead to health inequities (Curtis et al., 2012; LaVeist and Pierre, 2014). Identification of potential candidates for the health professions starts with secondary school recruitment, although efforts to build the pool of future candidates need to begin much earlier through community engagement activities (McKendall et al., 2014; Phillips and Malone, 2014; WHO, 2006). Curtis and colleagues (2012) describe the recruitment pipeline as beginning with early exposure of young students to health careers and enrichment activities that encourage academic achievement. Next is supporting students through transitions into and within health professional programs, as well as providing institutional, academic, and social assistance to retain students through graduation. Throughout the pipeline, professional workforce development that engages families and communities is particularly important during early exposure to career pathways. Across the entire pipeline are opportunities to involve communities, role models, and mentors in recruiting and retaining locally derived students and faculty from underrepresented communities to enhance workforce diversity and better address the needs and priorities of the communities they represent.

Workforce Diversity

In general, people stay within social networks that resemble their own sociodemographics (Freeman and Huang, 2014; McPherson et al., 2001). This tendency toward homophily results in homogeneous groups with similar backgrounds, cultures, attitudes, and opinions. Homophily has been shown to impact people's choices of whom to marry and befriend, as well as whom health professionals interact with at work, who collaborates on scientific research and publication, and who is hired (Freeman and Huang, 2014; Mascia et al., 2015; Maume, 2011; McPherson et al., 2001). As a result of closed social and occupational networks, positions are reinforced rather than challenged, which leads to greater group harmony with lower performance gains (Freeman and Huang, 2014; Phillips et al., 2009). For example, publications have been found to have greater impact when produced by a more ethnically diverse research group rather than a group with little to no diversity (Freeman and Huang, 2014). And exposure to multiple cultures correlates positively with enhanced creativity, provided individuals are open to other perspectives (Hoever et al., 2012; Leung et al., 2008).

Health professional schools are charged with the responsibility of preparing a competent health workforce that can meet the needs of a rapidly changing, racially and ethnically diverse population. Cultural competency training is a common strategy for creating a more culturally and linguistically competent health workforce (AHRQ, 2014). However, another, potentially more direct intervention is to recruit and retain faculty and health workers who reflect the cultural diversity of the community served (Anderson et al., 2003; Kreiner, 2009).

Recruitment and Retention

Having a diverse and inclusive faculty offers students and trainees of all backgrounds role models and mentors with life experiences and cultures similar to their own. However, recruiting and retaining minority and female faculty who themselves may feel unsupported can create barriers to achieving the desired mix of health professional educators, particularly in senior academic positions (Price et al., 2005; Smith et al., 2014; Whittaker et al., 2015). Phillips and Malone (2014) reviewed methods used to increase the racial and ethnic diversity in the nursing profession by recruiting and retaining underrepresented minority groups in undergraduate nursing programs. One of their recommendations is to establish "stronger linkages between nursing practice and the social determinants of health in nursing education and clinical practice" (p. 49). For increasing diversity in medicine, Nivet and Berlin (2014) recommend increasing the scope and effectiveness of pipeline programs to better ensure the success of minority and socioeconomically disadvantaged young people. They point to the successful Robert Wood Johnson Foundation Summer Medical and Dental Education Program, which cultivates local talent through personal as well as academic assistance (RWJF, 2011). Finally, as efforts are under way to assess and address the challenges to increasing the representation of minority students and faculty in the health professions, it is important to stress that successfully recruiting and sustaining a diverse academic workforce will require a shift in the institutional climate with respect to diversity (Butts et al., 2012; Price et al., 2009; Whittaker et al., 2015; Yager et al., 2007).

Recommendation

In reviewing the literature, the committee concluded that there remains a need for health professional schools and organizations to recruit and admit viable candidates from the pool of eligible[4] applicants who have been negatively affected by the social determinants of health. Equal emphasis on retaining these candidates once accepted into the program is essential. Candidates for student, trainee, and faculty positions will ideally be recruited from the local community and will represent the population to be served. In pursuit of this ideal, the committee puts forth the following recommendation:

> **Recommendation 2: To prepare health professionals to take action on the social determinants of health in, with, and across communities, health professional and educational associations and organizations at the global, regional, and national levels should apply the concepts embodied in the framework in partnering with communities to increase the inclusivity and diversity of the health professional student body and faculty.**

To enable action on this recommendation, health professional education and training institutions should support pipelines to higher education in the health professions in underserved communities, thus expanding the pool of viable candidates who have themselves been negatively affected by the social determinants of health.

ORGANIZATION

The Cambridge Dictionary defines "organization" as "a group of people who work together in an organized way for a shared purpose" (Cambridge University Press, 2016). Applying this definition within the context of this report, organizations include but are not limited to universities, schools, religious establishments, governmental and nongovernmental organizations, businesses, hospitals, and clinics.

High-level organizations—those that typically possess funds, prestige, or both—are positioned to set the tone for local organizations that have more direct contact with communities. For example, the call to action by government leaders following the World Conference on Social Determinants of Health that led to the Rio Declaration guided member states such as Canada to take local action to influence and improve the working and living conditions that affect the health and well-being of its citizens (PHAC, 2014). Similarly, national recognition of the need for greater diversity in

---

[4] The pool of eligible students starts with primary and secondary education to encourage a new generation of health workers who are at the pre-entry stage. It also includes adults who might enter the health workforce from other sectors, and current health workers looking to expand their knowledge or change their employment position.

nursing on the part of U.S. nursing organizations and government nursing divisions led to local initiatives focused on recruiting and retaining underrepresented minority groups in nursing education programs (Dapremont, 2012; Phillips and Malone, 2014).

Lessons learned from the work of Health Canada in promoting equity in the health sector point to the importance of a strong organizational culture for setting priorities to address the causes of disparities (PHAC, 2014). Key factors deemed necessary for initiating and sustaining action on activities addressing the social determinants of health include ethical, moral, and humanist commitments from leaders; well-resourced and -trained staff and partners; and supportive organizational environments (PHAC, 2014; Raphael et al., 2014) (see Box 4-4).

Vision for and Commitment to Education in the Social Determinants of Health

Health professional schools are part of the community they serve and have a unique opportunity to improve the community's living and working conditions. For example, academic institutions that engage local organizations and community members in offering career pathways to the health professions send a clear message about their commitment to addressing the social determinants of health within their community. And while expanding the diversity of students and faculty in health professional schools is critical, such efforts will have limited impact unless the climate of the institution goes beyond one of diversity to one of inclusivity (Nivet and Berlin, 2014). A culture of inclusivity moves organizations and institutions closer to desired transformative learning environments.

BOX 4-4
Components of the Organization Domain

Vision for and commitment to education in the social determinants of health
- Policies, strategies, and program reviews
- Resources
- Infrastructure
- Promotion/career pathways

Supportive organizational environment
- Transformative learning
- Dissemination of pedagogical research
- Faculty development/continuing professional development

Policies, Strategies, and Program Reviews

Integrating health equity into an organization's policies, strategies, and program reviews represents a significant step toward an institutional commitment to addressing the underlying causes of social disadvantage and marginalization (PHAC, 2014; PMAC Secretariat, 2014; Redwood-Campbell et al., 2011). To this end, the Health Resources and Services Administration's (HRSA's) Division of Nursing required its 2013 funding applicants to incorporate the social determinants of health into proposed strategies aimed at diversifying the nursing workforce to improve population health equity (Williams et al., 2014). The funding requirements included developing relevant measures and metrics so programs can be reviewed for their progress toward decreasing health disparities and improving health equity.

Resources

Often through research and grant-funded projects, health professional schools bring to bear financial resources for building partnerships between university and community organizations. The University of British Columbia provides multiple examples of context-specific work undertaken in partnership with community organizations (UBC, n.d.). In these examples, each group contributes unique resources that support mutually agreed-upon goals that benefit all the organizations involved.

Infrastructure and Promotion/Career Pathways

Effective community engagement requires strong commitment from faculty. However, few academic institutions invest in the infrastructure that can enable faculty members to work in and with communities (DiGirolamo et al., 2012; Gelmon et al., 2012; Nokes et al., 2013).

In 2012, a university working group was asked to recommend organizational structures that would better support, enhance, and deepen community engagement and community-engaged scholarship at the university. While the group noted a strong university commitment to community engagement, the existing organizational structures did not enable action on that commitment (UMASS Boston, 2014). The group determined that establishing a coordinating infrastructure to bring different parties together would better enable sustainable partnerships. The group also looked at evaluation of and rewards for faculty working in and with communities. The group, like others, found that the university had insufficient policies to support community engagement as core academic work (Ladhani et al., 2013; Michener et al., 2012; UMASS Boston, 2014).

Direct involvement of university leadership in the development of guide-lines for evaluating and rewarding community-engaged scholarship for ten-ure and promotion paths has been identified as a way of lowering barriers to greater community engagement in addressing the social determinants of health (Marrero et al., 2013). One example is the University of Minnesota, which recently revised its promotion and tenure guidelines to recognize com-munity engagement (Jordan et al., 2012). Others are making similar strides in this area (AAMC, 2002; Bringle et al., 2006; Loyola University Chicago, 2016; UMASS Boston, 2014; USF, 2016). In addition, the need for faculty release time to create, maintain, and sustain equitable partnerships that sometimes take years to cultivate could be factored into tenure decisions (Calleson et al., 2002; Nokes et al., 2013; Seifer et al., 2012).

Supportive Organizational Environment

Academic institutions that support transformative learning environ-ments take advantage of networking opportunities and partnerships for educating students, trainees, and health professionals (Frenk et al., 2010). Such an approach offers learners the opportunity to see and at times experi-ence the world from another's perspective. In addition, organizations that support experiential opportunities—a key part of transformative learning for addressing the social determinants of health—prepare students for work outside of the predictable environment of the university setting (Holland and Ramaley, 2008). Given the intractable nature of many older institu-tions of higher learning, small shifts toward transformative learning would represent large steps. More recently established health professional schools are arguably more malleable and have greater flexibility to support more proactive environments for transformative learning, and it would be ben-eficial to encourage them to do so.

Transformative Learning and Dissemination of Pedagogical Research

Understanding the comparative advantage of each organizational part-ner is a step toward developing a transformative approach to engage-ment that can advance both university and community goals (Holland and Ramaley, 2008). One study that examined the role of transformative learn-ing in cross-profession partnerships between campus faculty and county extension educators identified key factors in the success of such learning (Franz, 2002). Among other findings, the author states that a climate of independence mixed with interdependence is important for cross-profession relationship building and partnership formation. The author also asserts that "models of successful staff partnerships need to be identified and lauded across the organization." Communicating the value of transformative learning approaches for addressing the social determinants of health legitimizes interprofessional and cross-profession partnerships (Franz, 2002). Promoting and actively disseminating faculty research in this area by means of annual faculty reports, newsletters, and recognition of faculty excellence through chancellor's awards for distinguished scholarship, teaching, and service can diffuse such messages more broadly within and outside of universities (UMASS Boston, 2014).

Faculty Development/Continuing Professional Development

Academic institutions often provide faculty some form of support for training in teaching and research, but few provide development opportunities for community-engaged faculty members (Jordan et al., 2012). One exception is the University of Massachusetts' Civic Engagement Scholars Initiative within the university's Office for Faculty Development. This program supports faculty and departments engaged in redesigning and evaluating courses in the development of effective methods for engaging students in service-learning and community-based research activities that "reinforce classroom learning, foster civic habits and skills, and address community-identified needs" (Martinez-Krawiec, 2013).

Faculty development has been used as a tool for organizations seeking to recruit and retain a diverse workforce (Daley et al., 2006). The Office of Faculty Development at Harvard Medical School, for example, offers a comprehensive program that includes specific activities and events targeted at women and underrepresented minority faculty. Similarly, the Minority Faculty Leadership and Career Development Program at Boston University's Schools of Medicine and Public Health is a longitudinal leadership and career development program for underrepresented minority faculty (BUSM, 2015). Through self-reflection and assessment, experiential learning, and peer and senior mentorship, the program aims to provide faculty with tools to effect positive change throughout their careers.

Recommendation

The committee encourages organizations to build upon policies, strategies, programs, and structures already in place to transform learning environments such that they align with the framework presented in this report. A first step is to understand how the social determinants of health are reflected within the organization's founding and guiding policies, strategies, programs, and structures. Therefore, in response to the calls for action from signatories of the Rio Declaration, as well as many individual health professionals and their representative professional and educational organizations, the committee makes the following recommendation:

Recommendation 3: Governments and individual ministries (e.g., signatories of the Rio Declaration), health professional and educational associations and organizations, and community groups should foster an enabling environment that supports and values the integration of the framework's principles into their mission, culture, and work.

To accomplish this recommendation, national governments, individual ministries, and health professional and educational associations and organizations should review, map, and align their educational and professional vision, mission, and standards to include the social determinants of health as described in the framework. The following actions would demonstrate organizational support for enhancing competency for addressing the social determinants of health:

- Produce and effectively disseminate case studies and evaluations on the use of the framework, integrating lessons learned to build and strengthen work on health professional education in the social determinants of health.
- Work with relevant government bodies to support and promote health professional education in the social determinants of health by aligning policies, planning, and financing and investments.
- Introduce accreditation of health professional education where it does not exist and strengthen it where it does.
- Design and implement continuing professional development programs for faculty and teaching staff that promote health equity and are relevant to the evolving health and health care needs and priorities of local communities.
- Support experiential learning opportunities that are interprofessional and cross-sectoral and involve partnering with communities.

FITTING THE FRAMEWORK INTO A CONCEPTUAL MODEL

Anchoring the framework within a broader societal context can facilitate understanding and uptake of the framework. The committee's conceptual model (see Figure 4-2) draws on multiple sources to show how strengthening health professional education to address the social determinants of health can produce a competent health workforce able to partner with communities and other sectors to improve the socioeconomic and political conditions that lead to health inequity and diminish health and well-being (Frenk et al., 2010; HHS, 2010; Solar and Irwin, 2010; Sousa et al., 2013; WHO, 2006, 2008b, 2011b).

At the left of the committee's conceptual model is the *socioeconomic and political context*, broadly defined as including all social and political

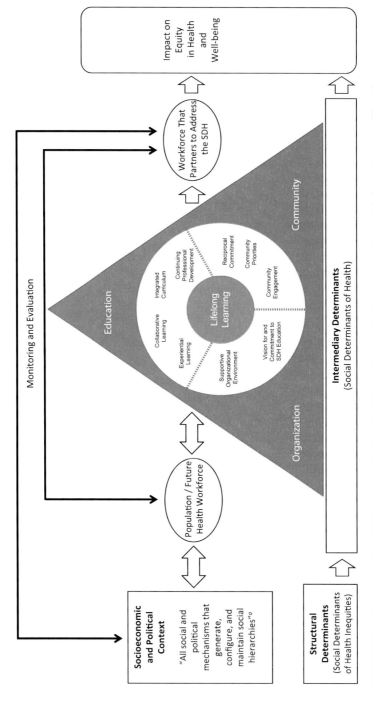

FIGURE 4-2 Conceptual model for strengthening health professional education in the social determinants of health.

NOTE: SDH = social determinants of health.

[a] Solar and Irwin, 2010, p. 5.

mechanisms that generate, configure, and maintain social hierarchies. These hierarchies are established through the labor market, the education system, political institutions, and societal and cultural values. Income, education, occupation, social class, gender, and race/ethnicity are the factors that stratify populations and lead to social hierarchies.

Context, structural mechanisms, and the resultant socioeconomic position of individuals are *structural determinants*, at the lower left of Figure 4-2, and in effect it is these determinants that are referred to as the *social determinants of health inequities*. The social determinants of health inequities operate through a set of *intermediary determinants* of health, shown at the bottom of the figure, to shape health outcomes. Intermediary determinants include material and psychosocial circumstances, behavioral and/or biological factors, and the health system (Solar and Irwin, 2010).

Positioned in the center of the model as an intermediary determinant is the committee's framework for lifelong learning for health professionals in understanding and addressing the social determinants of health. To the left of the framework is the *population/future health workforce*, which forms the pipeline for the education and production of future health professionals. Through the transformative learning approach described in the framework, health professionals, students, and trainees learn how to establish equal partnerships with communities, other sectors, and other professions for better understanding of and action on the social determinants of health. They also gain competency in addressing health system complexities within an increasingly global and interconnected world. The result is a *workforce that partners to address the social determinants of health* for the ultimate goal of an *impact on equity in health and well-being*.

The measurable output of the framework is a diverse and inclusive workforce that partners with other sectors, community organizations, community members, and other health professions to address and act on the social determinants of health. Monitoring and evaluation of this output would track progress on recruitment and retention of a diverse health professional student body and faculty that also mirrors local populations.

BUILDING THE EVIDENCE BASE

The committee's data collection and literature review efforts made clear that the impact on health professionals, students, and trainees of transformative learning that addresses the social determinants of health to effect the desired outcomes has not been well studied. And while the committee believes that such research would reveal positive impacts, there remains a relative lack of outcome research that goes beyond learning. Despite this research gap, promising educational practices and experiences reveal that community engagement—pursued in a respectful, informed, and sustainable manner—is critical to the effective education of health professionals in addressing the social determinants of health (Bainbridge et al., 2014; Feder et al., 2013). However, even lessons learned from educational experiences designed to impact the social determinants of health are not well articulated in the literature, nor are they widely disseminated. As a consequence, there remains a need to identify factors and processes that are common to promising practices and experiences to inform the education of health professionals in understanding and acting on the social determinants of health.

Such analyses would go beyond self-examination to include input from community partners to demonstrate objective and subjective impacts. These efforts would inform best practices for transformative learning. Given the need for evidence that learning in and with communities impacts the social determinants of health, the committee makes the following recommendation for building the evidence base:

> **Recommendation 4: Governments, health professional and educational associations and organizations, and community organizations should use the committee's framework and model to guide and support evaluation research aimed at identifying and illustrating effective approaches for learning about the social determinants of health in and with communities while improving health outcomes, thereby building the evidence base.**

To demonstrate full and equal partnerships, health professional and educational associations and organizations and community partners should prepare their respective networks to engage with one another in a systematic, comprehensive inquiry aimed at building the evidence base.

The committee also proposes an approach that, if undertaken, could provide strategic direction for efforts to build the evidence base in and with communities (see Box 4-5).

MOVING FORWARD

There are many challenges to educating health professionals to understand and act upon the social determinants of health in and with communities. Designing and instituting robust experiences is time-consuming for faculty and others. The process is labor-intensive and requires a strong commitment from the community, whose trust must be gained over time through demonstration of the value of partnerships. Such partnerships are not stagnant; rather, they must be flexible to evolve as community needs and desires change over time. The need for such flexibility can present difficulties for educators, who are often underresourced. Other challenges stem from learners themselves, who may be resistant to community experi-

---

BOX 4-5
Building the Evidence Base

Systematic, comprehensive inquiry should be undertaken to identify and illustrate effective approaches to

- creating a strategic planning process that involves all relevant partners critical to addressing the social determinants of health within the community of interest;
- assessing community readiness to partner with educational institutions and other organizations to determine relevant assets, needs, and commitment through asset mapping and needs analysis;
- undertaking community review of gaps, priorities, and assets for acquiring necessary resources;
- mobilizing key stakeholders within the community to secure resources and ensure stakeholders' commitment and participation;
- developing an infrastructure for organizing, deploying, and managing these resources;
- joining as well as initiating mechanisms for engaging educational institutions and other organizations;
- increasing human capital within the community to recognize, understand, and address the social determinants of health as they unfold within the lives of community members;
- ensuring constructive, continuous mechanisms for community review of processes and accomplishments;
- pursuing these objectives in a respectful, trusting manner that expects of others a similar approach to honoring these relationships;
- creating mechanisms for communicating in an ongoing, transparent fashion; and
- translating the results of these partnerships into advocacy and policy development.

---

ences that shift power from the learner or the provider to the community and its members. Finding faculty who understand and can offer effective learning opportunities that demonstrate how the social determinants of health impact individuals, populations, and communities poses an additional challenge.

Despite these challenges, the potential financial, social, and political returns from such an investment in education are great. The first is improved community relations. At a time of community distrust and turmoil, creating strong partnerships that demonstrate support over time could help ease tensions within communities. Second, community interventions could create pathways for young people from underperforming communities to enter the health professions and give back to their community as providers and role models for future generations. Third, health care providers and their students and trainees could become more effective clinicians by understanding the entire health system and how external economic, financial, and policy forces can impact the home, family, and community in which a patient resides. Fourth, by exposing learners to other professions and other sectors, working in the community could create a broader understanding of health systems and how interactions among partners are essential for impacting individual and population health outcomes, which in turn generates demonstrable cost savings for payers of health care. Finally, in a time of increasing globalization, migration, and mixing of cultures, building a workforce that can work in and with different communities could increase the effectiveness of early interventions that can improve quality of life while decreasing costs associated with interventions undertaken later on.

Support from multiple stakeholders at all levels will be necessary for these benefits to be realized. Garnering that support will require reaching beyond traditional health professional education pedagogy and silos and engaging new players, such as community health workers and other trusted members of the community, in equal partnership to address community concerns while educating health professionals (Johnson et al., 2012; Torres et al., 2014). Planning will also be necessary to engage nonhealth sectors such as education (e.g., at the primary and secondary levels), labor, housing, transportation, urban planning, community development, and public policy.

Financing has traditionally been an obstacle to offering robust opportunities for any of the components of the framework. Finding the necessary resources needs to start with a strong commitment from organizations and leaders based on the realization that without adequate and sustained funding, efforts toward transformative learning will remain predominantly one-off, ad hoc initiatives by motivated but often overburdened, undersupported individuals. Health professionals are in key positions to impact the social determinants of health if they act in a coordinated manner. A detailed description of the financing of health professional education is beyond this committee's charge; nonetheless, given the critical role of funding in fulfilling the vision of transformative learning set forth in this report, the committee believes it is important to make a few points on this topic.

First, governments and ministries are in a position to redirect incentives for real and sustained community engagement through funding mechanisms, special tax status, and educational requirements. Some governments, ministries, and foundations are also in a position to direct research support toward efforts to demonstrate the value of partnerships for improving certain indicators of success, such as financial savings and the health and well-being of communities across generations.

Second, anyone with a stake in how health professionals are educated and trained can become an advocate for experiential learning addressing the social determinants of health. As discussed in Chapter 1, many groups have called for action on the social determinants of health. Each such group can exert pressure to update curricula to better reflect the world in which health professionals are expected to work. Health professionals trained to be critical thinkers are better positioned to function effectively in today's world, in which they increasingly must work with others in and outside of the health system. With specific exposure and training in policy, even students and representatives from small organizations and institutions can play a role in advocating for changes in funding to support education that demonstrates value to communities. This advocacy might involve partnerships between community organizations and universities to establish or improve education pipelines so as to increase the representation of community members in education and the local health workforce.

Finally, to advocate effectively for change, it will be necessary to have population-based data demonstrating the value of investments in the education of health professionals in addressing the social determinants of health in and with communities to all stakeholders in terms of finances, health improvements, and quality of life. Despite even the best evidence, however, resistance to change is likely. Forcing a shift in education through accreditation standards could result in health professional education reflecting more of the framework components. However, to achieve transformative learning based on the framework that can create the envisioned systems thinkers and inspired lifelong learners about the social determinants of health, support for educators will be necessary. The lack of such support could result in lackluster or segmented course offerings related to the social determinants of health and even damage to community relations if learning institutions minimally complied with regulations. In this regard, educational leadership could be held accountable through policy and other reviews conducted by advocates such as students and faculty who understood the need for a new paradigm for learning about and acting on the social determinants of health.

In closing, the committee reiterates that passive learning is not sufficient to fully develop the competencies needed by health professionals to understand and address the social determinants of health. To impact health equity, health professionals need to translate knowledge to action, which requires more than accruing knowledge. Health professionals need to develop appropriate skills and attitudes to be advocates for change. Governments, ministries, communities, foundations, and health professional and educational associations all have a role in how health professionals learn to address the social determinants of health. Using the committee's framework and associated conceptual model as a guide, these groups can visualize how organizations, educational institutions and associations, and communities can come together to eliminate health inequities through collective actions. The realization of this vision begins with building a competent health workforce that is appropriately educated and trained to address the social determinants of health.

REFERENCES

AAMC (Association of American Medical Colleges). 2002. *The scholarship of community engagement: Using promotion and tenure guidelines to support faculty work in communities.* https://depts.washington.edu/ccph/pdf_files/AAMC.pdf (accessed September 22, 2016).

Abdulrahim, S., M. El Shareef, M. Alameddine, R. A. Afifi, and S. Hammad. 2010. The potentials and challenges of an academic-community partnership in a low-trust urban context. *Journal of Urban Health: Bulletin of the New York Academy of Medicine* 87(6):1017-1020.

AHRQ (Agency for Healthcare Research and Quality). 2014. *Evidence-based practice center systematic review protocol: Improving cultural competence to reduce health disparities for priority populations.* http://effectivehealthcare.ahrq.gov/ehc/products/573/1934/cultural-competence-protocol-140709.pdf (accessed September 22, 2016).

Anderson, E. S., R. Smith, and L. N. Thorpe. 2010. Learning from lives together: Medical and social work students' experiences of learning from people with disabilities in the community. *Health & Social Care in the Community* 18(3):229-240.

Anderson, L. M., S. C. Scrimshaw, M. T. Fullilove, J. E. Fielding, J. Normand, and the Task Force on Community Preventive Services. 2003. Culturally competent healthcare systems. A systematic review. *American Journal of Preventive Medicine* 24(Suppl. 3):68-79.

Art, B., L. De Roo, and J. De Maeseneer. 2007. Towards Unity for Health utilising community-oriented primary care in education and practice. *Education for Health (Abingdon, England)* 20(2):74.

Bainbridge, L., S. Grossman, S. Dharamsi, J. Porter, and V. Wood. 2014. Engagement studios: Students and communities working to address the determinants of health. *Education for Health (Abingdon, England)* 27(1):78-82.

Barman, A., R. Jaafar, and N. M. Ismail. 2006. Problem-based learning as perceived by dental students in Universiti Sains Malaysia. *Malaysian Journal of Medical Sciences* 13(1):63-67.

Berk, R. A. 2009. Using the 360 degrees multisource feedback model to evaluate teaching and professionalism. *Medical Teacher* 31(12):1073-1080.

Bhatia, R., L. Farhang, J. Heller, M. Lee, M. Orenstein, M. Richardson, and A. Wernham. 2014. *Minimum elements and practice standards for health impact assessment, version 3, September.* Oakland, CA: HIA Practice Standards Working Group.

Blumenthal, D. S. 2011. Is community-based participatory research possible? *American Journal of Preventive Medicine* 40(3):386-389.

Brauer, D. G., and K. J. Ferguson. 2015. The integrated curriculum in medical education: AMEE Guide No. 96. *Medical Teacher* 37(4):312-322.

Bringle, R. G., J. A. Hatcher, S. Jones, and W. M. Plater. 2006. Sustaining civic engagement: Faculty development, roles, and rewards. *Metropolitan Universities* 17(1):62-74.

Buckner, A. V., Y. D. Ndjakani, B. Banks, and D. S. Blumenthal. 2010. Using service-learning to teach community health: The Morehouse School of Medicine community health course. *Academic Medicine* 85(10):1645-1651.

Burnett, S. M., M. K. Mbonye, S. Naikoba, S. Zawedde-Muyanja, S. N. Kinoti, A. Ronald, T. Rubashembusya, K. S. Willis, R. Colebunders, Y. C. Manabe, and M. R. Weaver. 2015. Effect of educational outreach timing and duration on facility performance for infectious disease care in Uganda: A trial with pre-post and cluster randomized controlled components. *PLoS ONE* 10(9):e0136966.

BUSM (Boston University School of Medicine). 2015. *Minority Faculty Leadership & Career Development Program.* http://www.bumc.bu.edu/facdev-medicine/facdevprograms/minority-faculty-leadership-career-development-program (accessed September 22, 2016).

Butts, G. C., Y. Hurd, A. G. S. Palermo, D. Delbrune, S. Saran, C. Zony, and T. A. Krulwich. 2012. Role of institutional climate in fostering diversity in biomedical research workforce: A case study. *The Mount Sinai Journal of Medicine, New York* 79(4):498-511.

Caldron, P. H., A. Impens, M. Pavlova, and W. Groot. 2015. A systematic review of social, economic and diplomatic aspects of short-term medical missions. *BMC Health Services Research* 15:380.

Calleson, D. C., S. D. Seifer, and C. Maurana. 2002. Forces affecting community involvement of AHCS: Perspectives of institutional and faculty leaders. *Academic Medicine* 77(1):72-81.

Cambridge University Press. 2016. *Organization.* http://dictionary.cambridge.org/us/dictionary/english/organization (accessed May 31, 2016).

Campbell, C., K. Scott, M. Nhamo, C. Nyamukapa, C. Madanhire, M. Skovdal, L. Sherr, and S. Gregson. 2013a. Social capital and HIV competent communities: The role of community groups in managing HIV/AIDS in rural Zimbabwe. *AIDS Care* 25(Suppl. 1):S114-S122.

Campbell, C., M. Nhamo, K. Scott, C. Madanhire, C. Nyamukapa, M. Skovdal, and S. Gregson. 2013b. The role of community conversations in facilitating local HIV competence: Case study from rural Zimbabwe. *BMC Public Health* 13:354.

Carman, A. L. 2015. Collective impact through public health and academic partnerships: A Kentucky public health accreditation readiness example. *Frontiers in Public Health* 3:44.

Cashman, S., J. Hale, L. Candib, T. A. Nimiroski, and D. Brookings. 2004. Applying service-learning through a community-academic partnership: Depression screening at a federally funded community health center. *Education for Health (Abingdon, England)* 17(3):313-322.

Cené, C. W., M. E. Peek, E. Jacobs, and C. R. Horowitz. 2010. Community-based teaching about health disparities: Combining education, scholarship, and community service. *Journal of General Internal Medicine* 25 (Suppl 2.):S130-S135.

Chou, C. L., K. Hirschmann, A. H. Fortin VII, and P. R. Lichstein. 2014. The impact of a faculty learning community on professional and personal development: The facilitator training program of the American Academy on Communication in Healthcare. *Academic Medicine* 89(7):1051-1056.

Christopher, S., V. Watts, A. K. H. G. McCormick, and S. Young. 2008. Building and maintaining trust in a community-based participatory research partnership. *American Journal of Public Health* 98(8):1398-1406.

Collins, J., and J. Koplan. 2009. Health impact assessment: A step toward health in all policies. *Journal of the American Medical Association* 302(3):315-317.

Cónsul-Giribet, M., and J. L. Medina-Moya. 2014. Strengths and weaknesses of problem based learning from the professional perspective of registered nurses. *Revista Latino-Americana de Enfermagem* 22(5):724-730.

Council of the European Union. 2002. Council resolution of 27 June 2002 on lifelong learning. *Official Journal of the European Communities* C163/1-C163/3.

Curtis, E., E. Wikaire, K. Stokes, and P. Reid. 2012. Addressing indigenous health workforce inequities: A literature review exploring "best" practice for recruitment into tertiary health programmes. *International Journal for Equity in Health* 11:13.

Daley, S., D. L. Wingard, and V. Reznik. 2006. Improving the retention of underrepresented minority faculty in academic medicine. *Journal of the National Medical Association* 98(9):1435-1440.

Dapremont, J. A. 2012. A review of minority recruitment and retention models implemented in undergraduate nursing programs. *Journal of Nursing Education and Practice* 3(2):112-119.

DiGirolamo, A., A. C. Geller, S. A. Tendulkar, P. Patil, and K. Hacker. 2012. Community-based participatory research skills and training needs in a sample of academic researchers from a clinical and translational science center in the northeast. *Clinical and Translational Science* 5(3):301-305.

Dillenbourg, P. 1999. What do you mean by collaborative learning? In *Collaborative-learning: Cognitive and computational approaches*, edited by P. Dillenbourg. Oxford, UK: Elsevier. Pp. 1-19.

Donnon, T., A. Al Ansari, S. Al Alawi, and C. Violato. 2014. The reliability, validity, and feasibility of multisource feedback physician assessment: A systematic review. *Academic Medicine* 89(3):511-516.

Dooly, M. 2008. Constructing knowledge together. In *Telecollaborative language learning: A guidebook to moderating intercultural collaboration online*, edited by M. Dooly. Bern, NY: Peter Lang. Pp. 21-45.

Doran, K. M., K. Kirley, A. R. Barnosky, J. C. Williams, and J. E. Cheng. 2008. Developing a novel poverty in healthcare curriculum for medical students at the University of Michigan Medical School. *Academic Medicine* 83(1):5-13.

Economos, C. D., and S. Irish-Hauser. 2007. Community interventions: A brief overview and their application to the obesity epidemic. *Journal of Law, Medicine & Ethics* 35(1):131-137.

Edutopia. 2016. *Project-based learning.* http://www.edutopia.org/project-based-learning (accessed January 11, 2016).

El-Sayed, M., and J. El-Sayed. 2014. Achieving lifelong learning outcomes in professional degree programs. *International Journal of Process Education* 6(1):37-42.

Feder, E., C. Moran, A. Gargano Ahmed, S. Lessem, and R. Steidl. 2013. *Limiting retail alcohol outlets in the Greenbush-Vilas neighborhood, Madison, Wisconsin: A health impact assessment.* Madison, WI: University of Wisconsin Population Health Institute.

FIP (International Pharmaceutical Federation). 2014. *Continuing professional development/continuing education in pharmacy: Global report.* The Hague, The Netherlands: FIP.

Franz, N. K. 2002. *Transformative learning in extension staff partnerships: Facilitating personal, joint, and organizational change.* Paper presented at Annual Meeting of the Association for Leadership Education, Lexington, KY, July 11-13.

Freeman, R. B., and W. Huang. 2014. Collaboration: Strength in diversity. *Nature* 513(7518):305.

Frenk, J., L. Chen, Z. A. Bhutta, J. Cohen, N. Crisp, T. Evans, H. Fineberg, P. Garcia, Y. Ke, P. Kelley, B. Kistnasamy, A. Meleis, D. Naylor, A. Pablos-Mendez, S. Reddy, S. Scrimshaw, J. Sepulveda, D. Serwadda, and H. Zurayk. 2010. Health professionals for a new century: Transforming education to strengthen health systems in an interdependent world. *Lancet* 376(9756):1923-1958.

Frenk, J., D. J. Hunter, and I. Lapp. 2015. A renewed vision for higher education in public health. *American Journal of Public Health* 105(Suppl. 1):S109-S113.

Furco, A. 1996. Service-learning: A balanced approach to experiential education. In *Expanding boundaries: Serving and learning*, edited by B. Taylor and Corporation for National Service. Washington, DC: Corporation for National Service. Pp. 2-6.

Gelmon, S., K. Ryan, L. Blanchard, and S. D. Seifer. 2012. Building capacity for community-engaged scholarship: Evaluation of the faculty development component of the faculty for the engaged campus initiative. *Journal of Higher Education Outreach and Engagement* 16(1):21-45.

Goldberg-Freeman, C., N. E. Kass, P. Tracey, G. Ross, B. Bates-Hopkins, L. Purnell, B. Canniffe, and M. Farfel. 2007. "You've got to understand community": Community perceptions on "breaking the disconnect" between researchers and communities. *Progress in Community Health Partnerships* 1(3):231-240.

Heller, J., M. L. Givens, T. K. Yuen, S. Gould, M. B. Jandu, E. Bourcier, and T. Choi. 2014. Advancing efforts to achieve health equity: Equity metrics for health impact assessment practice. *International Journal of Environmental Research and Public Health* 11(11):11054-11064.

HHS (U.S. Department of Health and Human Services). 2010. *Healthy People 2020*. Washington, DC: HHS. http://www.healthypeople.gov/sites/default/files/HP2020_brochure_with_LHI_508_FNL.pdf (accessed January 11, 2016).

Hoever, I. J., D. van Knippenberg, W. P. van Ginkel, and H. G. Barkema. 2012. Fostering team creativity: Perspective taking as key to unlocking diversity's potential. *Journal of Applied Physiology* 97(5):982-996.

Holland, B., and J. A. Ramaley. 2008. *Creating a supportive environment for community-university engagement: Conceptual frameworks*. Sydney, New South Wales: Higher Education Research and Development Society of Australasia, Inc. (HERDSA).

Howard, K. M., T. Stewart, W. Woodall, K. Kingsley, and M. Ditmyer. 2009. An integrated curriculum: Evolution, evaluation, and future direction. *Journal of Dental Education* 73(8):962-971.

Hunt, J. B., C. Bonham, and L. Jones. 2011. Understanding the goals of service learning and community-based medical education: A systematic review. *Academic Medicine* 86(2):246-251.

Ivicek, K., A. B. de Castro, M. K. Salazar, H. H. Murphy, and M. Keifer. 2011. Using problem-based learning for occupational and environmental health nursing education: Pesticide exposures among migrant agricultural workers. *Journal of the American Association of Occupational Health Nurses* 59(3):127-133.

Jagosh, J., P. Bush, J. Salsberg, A. Macaulay, T. Greenhalgh, G. Wong, M. Cargo, L. Green, C. Herbert, and P. Pluye. 2015. A realist evaluation of community-based participatory research: Partnership synergy, trust building and related ripple effects. *BMC Public Health* 15(1):725.

Johnson, D., P. Saavedra, E. Sun, A. Stageman, D. Grovet, C. Alfero, C. Maynes, B. Skipper, W. Powell, and A. Kaufman. 2012. Community health workers and Medicaid managed care in New Mexico. *Journal of Community Health* 37(3):563-571.

Jordan, C., W. J. Doherty, R. Jones-Webb, N. Cook, G. Dubrow, and T. J. Mendenhall. 2012. Competency-based faculty development in community-engaged scholarship: A diffusion of innovation approach. *Journal of Higher Education Outreach and Engagement* 16(1):65-96.

Josiah Macy Jr. Foundation. 2010. *Lifelong learning in medicine and nursing: Final conference report*. New York: Josiah Macy Jr. Foundation. http://www.aacn.nche.edu/education-resources/MacyReport.pdf (accessed September 22, 2016).

Kelley, M. A., W. Baldyga, F. Barajas, and M. Rodriguez-Sanchez. 2005. Capturing change in a community-university partnership: The ¡sí se puede! Project. *Preventing Chronic Disease* 2(2):A22.

Khoiriyah, U., C. Roberts, C. Jorm, and C. P. M. Van der Vleuten. 2015. Enhancing students' learning in problem based learning: Validation of a self-assessment scale for active learning and critical thinking. *BMC Medical Education* 15:140.

Kickbusch, I. 2013. A game change in global health: The best is yet to come. *Public Health Reviews* 35(1).

Kitto, S., J. Goldman, M. H. Schmitt, and C. A. Olson. 2014. Examining the intersections between continuing education, interprofessional education and workplace learning. *Journal of Interprofessional Care* 28(3):183-185.

Kolb, D. A. 1984. *Experiential learning: Experience as the source of learning and development.* Englewood Cliffs, NJ: Prentice-Hall.

Kreiner, M. 2009. Delivering diversity: Newly regulated midwifery returns to Manitoba, Canada, one community at a time. *The Journal of Midwifery & Women's Health* 54(1):e1-e10.

Kretzmann, J. P., J. L. McKnight, S. Dobrowolski, D. Puntenney. 2005. *Discovering community power: A guide to mobilizing local assets and your organization's capacity.* Evanston, IL: Asset Based Community Development Institute, Northwestern University. http://www.abcdinstitute.org/docs/kelloggabcd.pdf (accessed September 22, 2016).

Ladhani, Z., F. J. Stevens, and A. J. Scherpbier. 2013. Competence, commitment and opportunity: An exploration of faculty views and perceptions on community-based education. *BMC Medical Education* 13(1):167.

Lane, E. A. 2008. Problem-based learning in veterinary education. *Journal of Veterinary Medical Education* 35(4):631-636.

Langlois, J. P., and S. B. Thach. 2003. Bringing faculty development to community-based preceptors. *Academic Medicine* 78(2):150-155.

LaVeist, T. A., and G. Pierre. 2014. Integrating the 3Ds-social determinants, health disparities, and health-care workforce diversity. *Public Health Reports-US* 129(Suppl. 2):9-14.

Lawlor, E. F., M. W. Kreuter, A. K. Sebert-Kuhlmann, and T. D. McBride. 2015. Methodological innovations in public health education: Transdisciplinary problem solving. *American Journal of Public Health* 105(Suppl. 1):S99-S103.

Leppo, K., E. Ollila, S. Peña, M. Wismar, and S. Cook. 2013. *Health in all policies: Seizing opportunities, implementing policies.* Helsinki, Finland: Ministry of Social Affairs and Health.

Leung, A. K., W. W. Maddux, A. D. Galinsky, and C. Y. Chiu. 2008. Multicultural experience enhances creativity: The when and how. *American Psychologist* 63(3):169-181.

Levy, M., D. Gentry, and L. M. Klesges. 2015. Innovations in public health education: Promoting professional development and a culture of health. *American Journal of Public Health* 105(Suppl. 1):S44-S45.

Lloyd, B., D. Pfeiffer, J. Dominish, G. Heading, D. Schmidt, and A. McCluskey. 2014. The new South Wales Allied Health Workplace Learning Study: Barriers and enablers to learning in the workplace. *BMC Health Services Research* 14(1):134.

Lomazzi, M., C. Jenkins, and B. Borisch. 2016. Global public health today: Connecting the dots. *Global Health Action* 9:28772.

Loyola University Chicago. 2016. *The scholarship of engagement.* http://www.luc.edu/experiential/engaged_scholars.shtml (accessed January 11, 2016).

Malik, R., R. Bordman, G. Regehr, and R. Freeman. 2007. Continuous quality improvement and community-based faculty development through an innovative site visit program at one institution. *Academic Medicine* 82(5):465-468.

Marrero, D. G., E. J. Hardwick, L. K. Staten, D. A. Savaiano, J. D. Odell, K. F. Comer, and C. Saha. 2013. Promotion and tenure for community engaged research: An examination of promotion and tenure support for community engaged research at three universities collaborating through a clinical and translational science award. *Clinical and Translational Science* 6(3):204-208.

Martinez-Krawiec, C. 2013. *Civic engagement scholars initiative (CESI)*. Paper 131. Boston, MA: Office of Community Partnerships Posters. http://scholarworks.umb.edu/ocp_posters/131 (accessed September 22, 2016).

Mascia, D., F. Di Vincenzo, V. Iacopino, M. P. Fantini, and A. Cicchetti. 2015. Unfolding similarity in interphysician networks: The impact of institutional and professional homophily. *BMC Health Services Research* 15:92.

Maume, D. J. 2011. Meet the new boss...Same as the old boss? Female supervisors and subordinate career prospects. *Social Science Research* 40(1):298.

McIntosh, S., R. C. Block, G. Kapsak, and T. A. Pearson. 2008. Training students in community health: A novel required fourth-year clerkship at the University of Rochester. *Academic Medicine* 83(4):357-364.

McKendall, S. B., K. Kasten, S. Hanks, and A. Chester. 2014. The Health Sciences and Technology Academy: An educational pipeline to address health care disparities in West Virginia. *Academic Medicine* 89(1):37-42.

McKnight, J. L., and J. P. Kretzmann. 1990. *Mapping community capacity*. Evanston, IL: Asset Based Community Development Institute, Northwestern University.

McLeroy, K. R., B. L. Norton, M. C. Kegler, J. N. Burdine, and C. V. Sumaya. 2003. Community-based interventions. *American Journal of Public Health* 93(4):529-533.

McNeil, R., M. Guirguis-Younger, L. B. Dilley, J. Turnbull, and S. W. Hwang. 2013. Learning to account for the social determinants of health affecting homeless persons. *Medical Education* 47(5):485-494.

McPherson, M., L. Smith-Loving, and J. M. Cook. 2001. Birds of a feather: Homophily in social networks. *Annual Review of Sociology* 27:415-444.

Metzler, M. M., D. L. Higgins, C. G. Beeker, N. Freudenberg, P. M. Lantz, K. D. Senturia, A. A. Eisinger, E. A. Viruell-Fuentes, B. Gheisar, A. G. Palermo, and D. Softley. 2003. Addressing urban health in Detroit, New York City, and Seattle through community-based participatory research partnerships. *American Journal of Public Health* 93(5):803-811.

Michener, L., J. Cook, S. M. Ahmed, M. A. Yonas, T. Coyne-Beasley, and S. Aguilar-Gaxiola. 2012. Aligning the goals of community-engaged research: Why and how academic health centers can successfully engage with communities to improve health. *Academic Medicine* 87(3):285-291.

Mihalynuk, T. V., P. Soule Odegard, R. Kang, M. Kedzierski, and N. Johnson Crowley. 2007. Partnering to enhance interprofessional service-learning innovations and addictions recovery. *Education for Health (Abingdon, England)* 20(3):92.

Mosavel, M., C. Simon, D. van Stade, and M. Buchbinder. 2005. Community-based participatory research (CBPR) in South Africa: Engaging multiple constituents to shape the research question. *Social Science & Medicine* 61(12):2577-2587.

Mulder, H., O. Ten Cate, R. Daalder, and J. Berkvens. 2010. Building a competency-based workplace curriculum around entrustable professional activities: The case of physician assistant training. *Medical Teacher* 32(10):e453-e459.

Murray, L. R., J. Garcia, M. Muñoz-Laboy, and R. G. Parker. 2011. Strange bedfellows: The Catholic Church and Brazilian National AIDS Program in the response to HIV/AIDS in Brazil. *Social Science & Medicine* 72(6):945-952.

Newman, P., and E. Peile. 2002. Learning in practice. Valuing learners' experience and supporting further growth: Educational models to help experienced adult learners in medicine. *British Medical Journal* 325:200-202.

NIH OBSSR (National Institutes of Health Office of Behavioral and Social Sciences Research). n.d. *Community-based participatory research*. https://obssr-archive.od.nih.gov/scientific_areas/methodology/community_based_participatory_research/index.aspx (accessed September 22, 2016).

Nisbet, G., M. Lincoln, and S. Dunn. 2013. Informal interprofessional learning: An untapped opportunity for learning and change within the workplace. *Journal of Interprofessional Care* 27(6):469-475.

Nivet, M. A., and A. Berlin. 2014. Workforce diversity and community-responsive health-care institutions. *Public Health Reports* 129(Suppl. 2):15-18.

Nokes, K. M., D. A. Nelson, M. A. McDonald, K. Hacker, J. Gosse, B. Sanford, and S. Opel. 2013. Faculty perceptions of how community-engaged research is valued in tenure, promotion and retention decisions. *Clinical and Translational Science* 6(4):259-266.

O'Sullivan, P. S., and D. M. Irby. 2011. Reframing research on faculty development. *Academic Medicine* 86(4):421-428.

Pearson, M. L., and H. T. Hubball. 2012. Curricular integration in pharmacy education. *American Journal of Pharmaceutical Education* 76(10):Article 204.

PHAC (Public Health Agency of Canada). 2014. *Toward health equity: Canadian approaches to the health sector pole.* Ottawa, ON: Public Health Agency of Canada.

Phillips, J. M., and B. Malone. 2014. Increasing racial/ethnic diversity in nursing to reduce health disparities and achieve health equity. *Public Health Reports* 129(Suppl. 2):45-50.

Phillips, K. W., K. A. Liljenquist, and M. A. Neale. 2009. Is the pain worth the gain? The advantages and liabilities of agreeing with socially distinct newcomers. *Personality and Social Psychology Bulletin* 35(3):336-350.

PMAC (Prince Mahidol Award Conference) Secretariat. 2014. Report on the 2014 conference on transformative learning for health equity: Prince Mahidol Award Conference 2014. Pattaya, Chonburi, Thailand. http://www.pmaconference.mahidol.ac.th/index.php?option=com_content&view=article&id=608&Itemid=207 (accessed June 2, 2016).

Price, E. G., A. Gozu, D. E. Kern, N. R. Powe, G. S. Wand, S. Golden, and L. A. Cooper. 2005. The role of cultural diversity climate in recruitment, promotion, and retention of faculty in academic medicine. *Journal of General Internal Medicine* 20(7):565-571.

Price, E. G., N. R. Powe, D. E. Kern, S. H. Golden, G. S. Wand, and L. A. Cooper. 2009. Improving the diversity climate in academic medicine: Faculty perceptions as a catalyst for institutional change. *Academic Medicine* 84(1):95-105.

Raphael, D., J. Brassolotto, and N. Baldeo. 2014. Ideological and organizational components of differing public health strategies for addressing the social determinants of health. *Health Promotion International* 1-13.

Redwood-Campbell, L., B. Pakes, K. Rouleau, C. J. MacDonald, N. Arya, E. Purkey, K. Schultz, R. Dhatt, B. Wilson, A. Hadi, and K. Pottie. 2011. Developing a curriculum framework for global health in family medicine: Emerging principles, competencies, and educational approaches. *BMC Medical Education* 11:46.

Regan-Smith, M. G. 1998. Teachers' experiential learning about learning. *International Journal of Psychiatry in Medicine* 28(1):11-20.

Rhodes, S. D., R. M. Malow, and C. Jolly. 2010. Community-based participatory research (CBPR): A new and not-so-new approach to HIV/AIDS prevention, care, and treatment. *AIDS Education and Prevention* 22(3):173-183.

Richmond, M., C. Canavan, M. C. Holtman, and P. J. Katsufrakis. 2011. Feasibility of implementing a standardized multisource feedback program in the graduate medical education environment. *Journal of Graduate Medical Education* 3(4):511-516.

Rock, J. A., J. M. Acuna, J. M. Lozano, I. L. Martinez, P. J. Greer, Jr., D. R. Brown, L. Brewster, and J. L. Simpson. 2014. Impact of an academic-community partnership in medical education on community health: Evaluation of a novel student-based home visitation program. *Southern Medical Journal* 107(4):203-211.

Ross, S. J., R. Preston, I. C. Lindemann, M. C. Matte, R. Samson, F. D. Tandinco, S. L. Larkins, B. Palsdottir, and A. J. Neusy. 2014. The training for health equity network evaluation framework: A pilot study at five health professional schools. *Education for Health (Abingdon, England)* 27(2):116-126.

RWJF (Robert Wood Johnson Foundation). 2011. *RWJF National Program report: Summer Medical and Dental Education Program.* http://www.rwjf.org/content/dam/farm/reports/program_results_reports/2013/rwjf70061 (accessed February 24, 2016).

Santilli, A., A. Carroll-Scott, F. Wong, and J. Ickovics. 2011. Urban youths go 3000 miles: Engaging and supporting young residents to conduct neighborhood asset mapping. *American Journal of Public Health* 101(12):2207-2210.

Schwartzman, R., and K. B. Henry. 2009. From celebration to critical investigation: Charting the course of scholarship in applied learning. *Journal of Applied Learning in Higher Education* 1:3-23.

Seifer, S. D., L. W. Blanchard, C. Jordan, S. Gelmon, and P. McGinley. 2012. Faculty for the engaged campus: Advancing community-engaged careers in the academy. *Journal of Higher Education Outreach and Engagement* 16(1):5-20.

Selamu, M., L. Asher, C. Hanlon, G. Medhin, M. Hailemariam, V. Patel, G. Thornicroft, and A. Fekadu. 2015. Beyond the biomedical: Community resources for mental health care in rural Ethiopia. *PLoS ONE* 10(5):e0126666.

Shreeve, M. W. 2008. Beyond the didactic classroom: Educational models to encourage active student involvement in learning. *The Journal of Chiropractic Education* 22(1):23-28.

Sigmon, R. 1979. Service-learning: Three principles. *Synergist. National Center for Service-Learning, ACTION* 8(1):9-11.

Smith, F., T. W. Lambert, and M. J. Goldacre. 2014. Demographic characteristics of doctors who intend to follow clinical academic careers: UK national questionnaire surveys. *Postgraduate Medical Journal* 90(1068):557-564.

Solar, O., and A. Irwin. 2010. *A conceptual framework for action on the social determinants of health. Social determinants of health discussion paper 2 (policy and practice).* Geneva, Switzerland: WHO. http://www.who.int/sdhconference/resources/ConceptualframeworkforactiononSDH_eng.pdf (accessed September 22, 2016).

Sousa, A., R. M. Scheffler, J. Nyoni, and T. Boerma. 2013. A comprehensive health labour market framework for universal health coverage. *Bulletin of the WHO* 91(11):892-894.

Strasser, R., P. Worley, F. Cristobal, D. C. Marsh, S. Berry, S. Strasser, and R. Ellaway. 2015. Putting communities in the driver's seat: The realities of community-engaged medical education. *Academic Medicine* 90(11):1466-1470.

Tan, E. J., S. McGill, E. K. Tanner, M. C. Carlson, G. W. Rebok, T. E. Seeman, and L. P. Fried. 2013. The evolution of an academic–community partnership in the design, implementation, and evaluation of Experience Corps® Baltimore city: A courtship model. *The Gerontologist* 54(2):314-321.

Taylor, I., and P. Le Riche. 2006. What do we know about partnership with service users and carers in social work education and how robust is the evidence base? *Health & Social Care in the Community* 14(5):418-425.

Teufel-Shone, N. I., T. Siyuja, H. J. Watahomigie, and S. Irwin. 2006. Community-based participatory research: Conducting a formative assessment of factors that influence youth wellness in the Hualapai community. *American Journal of Public Health* 96(9):1623-1628.

Thistlethwaite, J. E., E. Bartle, A. A. Chong, M. L. Dick, D. King, S. Mahoney, T. Papinczak, and G. Tucker. 2013. A review of longitudinal community and hospital placements in medical education: BEME Guide No. 26. *Medical Teacher* 35(8):e1340-e1364.

Thomas, J. W. 2000. *A review of research on project-based learning. Report prepared for the Autodesk Foundation.* http://www.bobpearlman.org/BestPractices/PBL_Research.pdf (accessed September 22, 2016).

Torres, S., R. Labonté, D. L. Spitzer, C. Andrew, and C. Amaratunga. 2014. Improving health equity: The promising role of community health workers in Canada. *Healthcare Policy* 10(1):73-85.

UBC (University of British Columbia). n.d. *Principles of community engagement: Resources and examples.* http://communityengagement.ubc.ca/scholarly-resources/principles-of-community-engagement-resources-and-examples (accessed September 22, 2016).

UMASS Boston (University of Massachusetts Boston). 2014. *Advancing community engaged scholarship and community engagement at the University of Massachusetts Boston: A report of the working group for an urban research-based action initiative.* Boston, MA: UMASS Boston. https://www.umb.edu/editor_uploads/images/research/Report_on_Community_Engaged_Scholarship.pdf (accessed September 22, 2016).

USF (University of South Florida). 2016. *Faculty: Tenure and promotion.* http://www.usf.edu/engagement/faculty/tenure-and-promotion.aspx (accessed January 11, 2016).

Wahab, M. S. A., R. A. J. Saad, and M. H. Selamat. 2014. A survey of work environment inhibitors to informal workplace learning activities amongst Malaysian accountants. In International Conference on Accounting Studies 2014, 18-19 August 2014, Kuala Lumpur, Malaysia, edited by K. I. Dandago, A. Che-Ahmad, A. Ahmi and S. Z. Saidin. Kuala Lumpur, Malaysia: *Procedia - Social and Behavioral Sciences* 164:409-414.

Wallerstein, N., and B. Duran. 2010. Community-based participatory research contributions to intervention research: The intersection of science and practice to improve health equity. *American Journal of Public Health* 100(Suppl. 1):S40-S46.

Walsh, A. 2005. *The tutor in problem based learning: A novice's guide.* Hamilton, ON: McMaster University. http://fhs.mcmaster.ca/facdev/documents/tutorPBL.pdf (accessed September 22, 2016).

Whittaker, J. A., B. L. Montgomery, and V. G. Martinez Acosta. 2015. Retention of under-represented minority faculty: Strategic initiatives for institutional value proposition based on perspectives from a range of academic institutions. *Journal of Undergraduate Neuroscience Education* 13(3):A136-A145.

WHO (World Health Organization). 2006. *The World Health Report 2006: Working together for health.* Geneva, Switzerland: WHO.

WHO. 2008a. *The World Health Report 2008. Primary health care: Now more than ever.* Geneva, Switzerland: WHO.

WHO. 2008b. *Closing the gap in a generation: Health equity through action on the social determinants of health, final report.* Geneva, Switzerland: WHO Commission on Social Determinants of Health.

WHO. 2011a. *Health systems strengthening glossary.* http://www.who.int/healthsystems/hss_glossary/en (accessed September 22, 2016).

WHO. 2011b. *Rio political declaration on social determinants of health.* Adopted at the World Conference on the Social Determinants of Health, Rio de Janeiro, Brazil. Geneva, Switzerland: WHO. http://www.who.int/sdhconference/declaration/Rio_political_declaration.pdf?ua=1 (accessed September 22, 2016).

WHO European Centre for Health Policy. 1999. *Gothenburg consensus paper. Health impact assessment: Main concepts and suggested approach.* Brussels, Belgium: European Centre for Health Policy. http://www.apho.org.uk/resource/item.aspx?RID=44163 (accessed September 22, 2016).

Williams, R. L., B. M. Shelley, and A. L. Sussman. 2009. The marriage of community-based participatory research and practice-based research networks: Can it work? -a research involving outpatient settings network (RIOS NET) study. *Journal of the American Board of Family Medicine* 22(4):428-435.

Williams, S. D., K. Hansen, M. Smithey, J. Burnley, M. Koplitz, K. Koyama, J. Young, and A. Bakos. 2014. Using social determinants of health to link health workforce diversity, care quality and access, and health disparities to achieve health equity in nursing. *Public Health Reports* 129(2):32-36.

Wilson, N. J., and R. Cordier. 2013. A narrative review of Men's Sheds literature: Reducing social isolation and promoting men's health and well-being. *Health & Social Care in the Community* 21(5):451-463.

Wood, D. F. 2003. Problem based learning. *British Medical Journal* 326(7384):328-330.

Yager, J., H. Waitzkin, T. Parker, and B. Duran. 2007. Educating, training, and mentoring minority faculty and other trainees in mental health services research. *Academic Psychiatry* 31(2):146-151.

Yang, J. 2015. *Recognition, validation and accreditation of non-formal and informal learning in UNESCO member states.* Hamburg, Germany: UNESCO Institute for Lifelong Learning. http://unesdoc.unesco.org/images/0023/002326/232656e.pdf (accessed September 22, 2016).

Appendix A

Educating Health Professionals to Address the Social Determinants of Health

Sara Willems, Ph.D., M.Sc.
Kaatje Van Roy, Ph.D., M.D., M.Sc.
Jan De Maeseneer, Ph.D., M.D.

INTRODUCTION

In 2015, the Institute of Medicine (IOM) convened a committee on educating health professionals to address the social determinants of health. A thorough search of the literature was needed in order for the committee to respond to its statement of task. This paper provides a review of the literature that describes the current practice of educating health professionals to address the social determinants of health in and with communities. Based on these findings, we formulate recommendations on how to strengthen health professional education by addressing the social determinants of health.

METHODS

Data Search

For this study, the Research Library of the National Academies of Sciences, Engineering, and Medicine conducted a literature search using the following databases: Medline, Cochrane Database of Systematic Reviews, Embase, Proquest, PubMed, Scopus, and Web of Science. The search terms were developed by IOM staff and study consultants. These search terms can be grouped into three categories: terms related to *primary social determinants*, to *health professions*, and to *education/learning* (see Box A-1).

The date range for the literature search was from 2000 to the present. Both U.S. and international materials were examined. Classroom and

---

BOX A-1
Overview of Search Terms

Social terms related to Primary Social Determinants
- Cultural Competence
- Cultural Competency
- Cultural Humility
- Social Determinants
- Social Determinants of Health
- Structural Violence
- Syndemics

Search terms related to Health Profession
- Health Professions Education
- Health Professional Education
- Continuing Professional Development
- Interprofessional Education

Search terms related to Education/Learning
- Service Learning
- Experiential Learning
- Problem Based Learning (Medical Subject Heading term for Experiential Learning)
- Community-Based Learning
- Community-Based Education
- Interprofessional Education

---

technology education were excluded from the search. The search was conducted between July 9 and July 14, 2015. This initial database search resulted in 297 papers. A team at the Department of Family Medicine and Primary Health Care of Ghent University then conducted an analysis of the identified papers. The team consisted of Sara Willems, master in health promotion and professor in health equity; Kaatje Van Roy, medical doctor, psychologist, and senior researcher; and Jan De Maeseneer, medical doctor, full professor in family medicine, and head of the department.

The team added four papers to the literature review, based on recommendations of consulted experts. Next, all papers were screened using the following inclusion criteria:

- The paper describes a training program for health care students or professionals.
- The described training program includes some form of experiential learning outside the classroom.

- The description of the learning aims, content, or outcome of the program refers to social determinants of health.

The screening was done independently by two researchers and in case of a different score, the paper was discussed until consensus was reached.

A first screening, based on titles and abstracts, resulted in the exclusion of 100 papers. During a second screening phase based on the full text of the remaining papers, another 168 papers were excluded. This two-phase screening process finally resulted in 33 papers being included in this review (see Figure A-1).

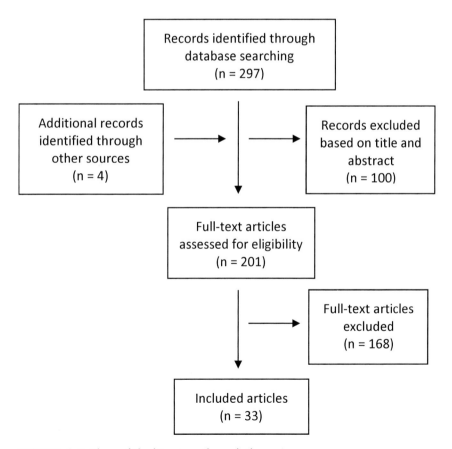

FIGURE A-1 Flow of the literature through the review.

Data Analysis

In line with the research questions of the present study, we designed an analytic instrument that allowed us to extract relevant information from each of the papers in a systematic way. This screening instrument allowed us to categorize the papers in terms of type of paper (e.g., research paper versus descriptive paper) and to extract details about the training program (e.g., duration of the training, the type of community that was involved in the program, information about the participants, the goal and the content of the program, the theoretical framework and pedagogical approach that were used). For the research papers, we also extracted information on the research aim, the method that was used, the number of participants, relevant findings for the present study, etc. The screening tool can be found in Annex A-1 at the end of this appendix.

RESULTS

Global Descriptions of the Programs

Location of the Schools Where the Programs Run

As noted, 33 papers describing training programs for health professional students addressing the social determinants of health in/with the community were found. Two papers reported on programs of the same school. The vast majority of the programs are from the United States (n = 24). The other schools are located in Canada (n = 6), Australia (n = 1), Belgium (n = 1), and Serbia (n = 1).

Type of Students for Which the Program Was Designed

Type of health profession Most programs are designed for medical (n = 10) and nursing (n = 8) students. Other included programs address pharmacy (n = 2), nurse practitioner (n = 1), physician assistant (n = 1), dentistry (n = 1), and art therapy students (n = 1). A considerable number of programs simultaneously involve students from different disciplines, including, for instance, medical, nursing, social work, and/or law students (n = 7). In these mixed groups, interprofessional learning often is an explicit learning objective.

Level Programs aim at students of different levels of training, including undergraduate, graduate, and doctoral. One program provides training to a mix of student levels; the service-learning program at the University of Arizona requires master's students to complete one course among five, whereas Ph.D. students are required to complete two of the five (option-ally one in co-teaching) (Sabo et al., 2015). Although none of the included programs was designed for health professionals, some programs were de-signed for students who already had some professional experience, such as registered nurse (R.N.)/bachelor of science in nursing (B.S.N.) students (Ezeonwu et al., 2014). Because of differences in terminology used (e.g., "undergraduate," "postbaccalaureate," "senior-level traditional students"), it sometimes proved difficult to evaluate the students' level.

Place of the Program in the Curriculum

While some programs are an obligatory component of the curriculum, others are elective or even extracurricular. In a limited number of cases, only selected students can attend the program. The selection procedure often comprises a written application exploring students' interests, previous experiences, and professional goals, sometimes combined with an interview (e.g., Bakshi et al., 2015; Kassam et al., 2013; Meili et al., 2011).

Length and Intensity of the Training

Programs largely vary with regard to their length and intensity. Pro-gram lengths range from approximately 1 week (e.g., Art et al., 2008), to over one semester (e.g., Bell and Buelow, 2014) to several years (e.g., Meurer et al., 2011). Furthermore, some of the programs are very intense (e.g., full-time presence in a community during an immersion experience abroad [Kassam et al., 2013; Meili et al., 2011]), while some are much less so (e.g., 1 hour per week [Kelly, 2013]). However, because of a lack of information, it is often difficult to get an encompassing idea of a program's extent. Moreover, programs vary in the amount of time dedicated to expe-riential learning versus time that is preserved for nonexperiential learning (more information on course content is provided below).

Communities Involved in the Training

Local communities In most programs, students have learning experiences in local communities. Community agencies and care providers that are involved in the programs comprise homeless shelters, domestic violence shelters, community health centers, schools, AIDS support organizations, substance abuse recovery centers, elderly homes, humanitarian organiza-tions, free clinics, and others. Correspondingly, students work with a large variety of populations, such as low-income populations, homeless people, native populations, migrant populations, and ethnic minority groups.

Communities abroad Some of the included programs provide international experiences to students. These include, for instance, a 6-week immersion in an AIDS support organization in Uganda (Kassam et al., 2013) and a 2-week stay at an indigenous Mayan community in Guatemala (Larson et al., 2010). One of the programs offers highly comprehensive training, including a 6-week stay in an Aboriginal community, a long-term engagement at an urban student-run clinic, and a 6-week stay at a rural hospital in Mozambique (Meili et al., 2011).

Theoretical Framework and Program Goals

Theoretical Framework

Programs are rooted within theoretical frameworks to various extents. Examples of such frameworks include cultural competence, social justice, social responsibility, social accountability, human rights, patient-centered care, and advocacy for patient health.

Program Goals

In many of the included papers, the program goals are more or less clearly stated. However, the extent to which these goals include learning about social determinants of health in an explicit way varies among the papers. Four types of goals were identified:

- The goals explicitly mention the social determinants of health (n = 9) (e.g., "to foster a better understanding of social determinants of health and ways of addressing health disparities" [Dharamsi et al., 2010a]).
- The goals mention health inequity or health disparities (n = 11) (e.g., "to provide the students the skills to plan, implement and evaluate a health disparity project" [Parks et al., 2015]).
- The goals implicitly refer to the social determinants of health (n = 12) (e.g., "to enhance students' knowledge and understanding of health issues and healthcare practice in rural and underserved communities" [Clithero et al., 2013]).
- Learning about the social determinants of health is not mentioned in the program goals, but appears to be an effect of the program (n = 1) (e.g., "It is evident that the nursing student learned about the influence of poverty on the health of children" [Ogenchuk et al., 2014]).

Some programs do not only define general learning goals but also require the students to outline some individual learning objectives (e.g., Brown et al., 2007; Meurer et al., 2011).

Pedagogical/Educational Approaches

Given the specific inclusion criteria that were used, learning approaches that do not include an experiential component in or with a community were excluded. "Service learning" appeared to be the most commonly used term in the included papers (at times combined with qualifier, as in "community service learning" or "international service learning"). In some papers, the authors provide background information about the way "service learning" is understood. The most commonly encountered understanding of service learning is presented in Box A-2. Another closely related term is "community-based learning." Other programs (additionally) focus on "interprofessional learning" or "interdisciplinary learning," in which different types of health students must work together. Less frequently encountered approaches include "community-oriented primary care" (e.g., Art et al., 2008) and "community-based participatory research" (e.g., Parks et al., 2015). Finally, there are some differences with regard to the setting in which learning takes place. Most often, the students spend time working in and with communities. A different approach is student-run clinics that provide health services to underserved neighborhoods or communities (Meili et al., 2011; Sheu et al., 2012).

BOX A-2
Service Learning

Numerous definitions of service learning are available. A definition that is often referred to is the one formulated by Health Professions Schools in Service to the Nation, outlining service learning as "a structured learning experience that combines community service with explicit learning objectives, preparation, and reflection" (Seifer, 1998, p. 274). This definition stresses the crucial components of service learning:

- Student learning should take place (allowing students to apply what they are learning to real-world situations).
- Community service and partnership take place (service learning is developed, implemented, and evaluated in collaboration with the community and responds to community-identified concerns).
- Opportunities for critical reflection are offered.

Program Components

The actual learning experience in the community can take various forms. Often-encountered components include conducting community (health) needs assessment, developing and implementing a project or intervention, organizing educational sessions for community members, and caring for individual patients.

Community needs assessment can be conducted through observation, windshield surveys, a review of demographic and health statistics, interviews with key informants, or focus groups with community members (e.g., Art et al., 2008; Dharamsi et al., 2010a; Ezeonwu et al., 2014; Kruger et al., 2010). Such needs assessment often serves as a first step in a community service learning project. After identifying the community needs, students gather further information and develop—in close collaboration with local community workers—a project that could counter one of these needs (e.g., Dharamsi et al., 2010a; Ezeonwu et al., 2014).

Teaching and interaction with community members are also often part of the program. In some programs, students organize health education sessions for the community members addressing different health-related topics (e.g., Bell and Buelow, 2014; Jarrell et al., 2014; Stanley, 2013; Ward et al., 2007). Getting to know community members and their living conditions includes, for instance, home visits (Art et al., 2008; De Los Santos et al., 2014), reading with children (Kelly, 2013), or art therapy students visiting a shelter for homeless persons and finding out what can be done with the children (Feen-Calligan, 2008). In an international learning experience with indigenous Mayan communities (Larson et al., 2010), students are lodged with families, often confronting daily life issues. One of the programs includes a component called "My Patient," in which the student follows a patient through his or her contacts with health care services and other health institutions and family settings. After each such visit, the student interviews the patient for at least 45 minutes (Matejic et al., 2012).

Taking care of individual community members is another component of some programs. Care for individual community members includes, for instance, home visits that focus on health education, arrangement of referrals, evaluation and improvement of health literacy, and development of an interprofessional care plan (De Los Santos et al., 2014). In some programs, a specific household or family is followed up by a student or an interprofessional group of students (e.g., De Los Santos et al., 2014; Ward et al., 2007). The Interprofessional Patient Advocacy course (Bell and Buelow, 2014) includes patient advocacy work ranging from helping patients complete applications or recertifications for Medicaid, housing, food stamps, or child care benefits; to providing support to patients with chronic conditions; to assisting in setting up health programs. Another way students carry out their health advocacy role is, for instance, writing a letter to the editor (Dharamsi et al., 2010a) or presenting survey findings to local key decision makers (Clithero et al., 2013). Profession-related care can also be part of the program. Examples include taking health histories, assisting local physicians with health assessments (Larson et al., 2010), providing foot care to persons in a homeless shelter (Schoon et al., 2012), and filling prescriptions or counseling patients (Brown et al., 2007). Learning to take care of patients and the community can also consist of shadowing a local community physician (Clithero et al., 2013; Kassam et al., 2013).

Sometimes, the experience is integrated into an already existing part of the curriculum. Sharma (2014), for example, describes a program that is integrated into medical residency training. Basically, the program incorporates reflection on the social determinants of health in the residents' daily work. For instance, the morning briefing is seen as a daily opportunity for discussion of root causes of ill health and is followed by an online blog. Moreover, during daily noon presentations, three additional questions are introduced systematically: (1) How do the social determinants of health pertain to your topic?, (2) How are certain groups at increased risk?, and (3) What are advocacy opportunities for physicians at the clinical or policy level?

In several programs, the experiential learning component is embedded in a broad approach that encompasses lectures, group discussions, workshops to build capacities (Dharamsi et al., 2010a), simulation experiences,[1] reading assignments,[2] online activities, including discussion fora with peers (e.g., Ezeonwu et al., 2014), presentations (e.g., Bell and Buelow, 2014; Ezeonwu et al., 2014), networking with alumni to promote project and career development (Williams et al., 2012), and research projects (e.g., Bakshi et al., 2015; Mudarikwa et al., 2010; Parks et al., 2015).

Reflective Learning

Personal reflection activities appear to be part of several programs. Several authors emphasize reflection as an indispensable component of true learning (e.g., Brown et al., 2007). According to Kelly (2013, p. 33), "the reflection piece truly separates service learning from volunteerism." Other authors draw attention to the fact that exposure alone does not guarantee better understanding and may even reinforce prejudice and stereotypes. Ezeonwu and colleagues (2014, p. 278) state that "it is the quality of reflection—thinking about the complex health care issues and using real life experiences to suggest questions for further exploration that transforms service into service

---

[1] Examples include an online poverty simulation (Bell and Buelow, 2014) and assessing barriers by stepping into the patient's role (Bussey-Jones et al., 2014).

[2] Actual examples of reading assignment texts are provided in Clithero et al. (2013).

learning." This is also confirmed by students stating that "the process of critical reflection is key to learning" (Dharamsi et al., 2010b). And by analyzing students' clinical journals, Bell and Buelow (2014) found that patient interactions often were only the start of learning, and that later self-reflection produced a more compelling understanding of the impact of poverty.

Reflection can be achieved in different ways. The range of reflective exercises includes

- keeping a daily reflective journal during the service experience;
- writing a report at the end of the experience;
- preparing a presentation for the trainers, community partners, and/ or fellow students;
- discussing with peers face-to-face or on an online forum; and
- photo-journaling.

In some cases, reflection is facilitated by the use of guiding questions (Ogenchuk et al., 2014), instruction to write on structured topics (see Box A-3), or use of the "critical incident technique" (Dharamsi et al., 2010a). Of interest, Kelly (2013, p. 33) notes that for true service learning, (medical) students need to be placed in an experience that is not part of their discipline, "as it allows students to set aside their medical skill sets and knowledge and genuinely focus on the community and the community issues."

BOX A-3
Examples of Topics Guiding Students' Reflection

1) Describe a situation which was complex, surprising, uncomfortable or uncertain using all five senses. Address your own biases and/or prejudices by reframing the encounter from a different point of view AFTER you have described it.
2) What interests you about this community/practice? What seems important?
3) What do you feel you are learning about medicine and about yourself?
4) Other-student choice. For example
   a) encounters with patients, colleagues, mentors
   b) questions about the patients you are seeing
   c) feelings about being in this particular community at this particular time in this particular way
   d) what is easy, difficult, puzzling, enjoyable, confusing, profound, boring, or rewarding about your experiences?

SOURCE: Excerpted from Clithero et al., 2013, p. 168.

Evaluation and Outcomes of the Programs

Many papers include some sort of evaluation of the program they describe. Such evaluation is obtained by means of quantitative data (n = 4), qualitative data (n = 7), a mix of qualitative and quantitative data (n = 9), or a rather informal and nonsystematic process (n = 8). Quantitative data basically rely on surveys measuring students' evaluation of and satisfaction with different aspects of the training, their career choices or readiness for inter-professional learning, and their attitudes toward the specific population with which they worked.[3] Qualitative data comprise mainly information obtained from students' reflective journals, focus groups, and interviews (most often with students, sometimes with trainers or community members). The impact of the program on students' identity, attitudes, cultural competence, etc., is the most prevalent type of qualitative data. Informal and nonsystematic evaluations stem principally from students' reflective journals and debriefing sessions. Generally, most such data are self-reported (students being asked about their own changes in attitudes or perceptions).

Students' Attitudes, Awareness, Understanding, and Skills

Frequently, students' awareness and understanding of the social determinants of health had deepened after the learning experience (e.g., Brown et al., 2007; Loewenson and Hunt, 2011; Schoon et al., 2012). They were able to see the bigger picture (Kruger et al., 2010), became aware of the impact of a lack of resources (Jarrell et al., 2014), and gained more insight into the complexity of the daily reality of community members (e.g., Meili et al., 2011).[4] Others bore witness to the fact that abstract concepts had turned into real experiences (Dharamsi et al., 2010b; Meili et al., 2011), as illustrated by this quote from one student: "Had you asked me before this experience what community health is I would have given you a definition. If you ask me now, I'll give you names, stories, laughs, somberness and actions" (Meili et al., 2011, p. 4). Students also acquired a better apperception of their future role as a health professional (Kruger et al., 2010).

Along with increased awareness and understanding, the learning experience affected students' attitudes at times. For instance, students showed more positive and nonstigmatizing attitudes toward homeless individuals after participating in structured clinical service-learning rotations with

---

[3] For example, Medical Student Attitudes Toward the Underserved (MSATU) (Bussey-Jones et al., 2014), Attitudes Toward Homelessness Inventory (ATHI) (Loewenson and Hunt, 2011), Belief in a Just World Scale (JWS), and Attitudes about Poverty and Poor People Scale (APPPS) (Jarrell et al., 2014).

[4] For example, by observing the distances the community members need to travel for appropriate health care (Meili et al., 2011).

homeless persons, and reported stronger beliefs, in the potential for viable programs or solutions to address homelessness (Loewenson and Hunt, 2011). Students also challenged their own stereotypes (Dharamsi et al., 2010b), beliefs, and attitudes with regard to the vulnerable populations with which they worked and discovered how much these people "were just like them" (Rasmor et al., 2014; Stanley, 2013). This was in contrast with the findings of another study that service learning can increase students' empathy toward those who live in poverty while at the same time solidifying perceptions that the poor are different from other members of society (Jarrell et al., 2014). Moreover, changes reported in the papers using quantitative analysis often are not statistically significant (e.g., Clithero et al., 2013; Jarrell et al., 2014; Rasmor et al., 2014; Sheu et al., 2012), so that solid conclusions on the actual effect of the training are difficult to draw.

After the learning experience, students often felt increased comfort in working with specific communities (Brown et al., 2007; Dharamsi et al., 2010a; Ierardi and Goldberg, 2014; Loewenson and Hunt, 2011). Gaining an understanding of the social determinants of health also helped the participants advocate for patients from vulnerable populations (Bakshi et al., 2015).

Interprofessionalism

The training programs that focused on interprofessionalism or interdisciplinarity often achieved their goals: students valued the interdisciplinary work (Art et al., 2008; Ierardi and Goldberg, 2014) and felt more ready for interprofessional learning (Sheu et al., 2012). Moreover, students learned that interdisciplinarity is important in a context of constrained resources (i.e., collaboration is all the more important when the number of professionals is limited) (Meili et al., 2011). Furthermore, O'Brien and colleagues (2014) note that the diversity of students provided a rich experiential base that contributed to monthly reflection sessions.

Long-Term Effects

In several cases, the training had an actual impact on students' career choices. Programs sometimes appeared to shape the students' desire to work with underserved populations (Dharamsi et al., 2010a; Meili et al., 2011; O'Brien et al., 2014), although students' preparedness to contribute to community-based volunteer activities in the future did not always change (Rasmor et al., 2014). Dharamsi and colleagues (2010a) also mention student-reported barriers, such as time limitations and financial obligations. Apart from one study in which students were interviewed 3 or 4 years after the learning experience (Ierardi and Goldberg, 2014), actual long-term effects could not be assessed, as data were most often gathered immediately after the training.

Most Valued Components

Some papers describe the components students valued most. Students often expressed their preference for interactive, community-based sessions over classroom didactics (Clithero et al., 2013; Meurer et al., 2011), claiming that they were learning more through the former (O'Brien et al., 2014). Students stressed the importance of witnessing and confrontations (Dharamsi et al., 2010a). Among the highest-rated course components for helping to understand their future role as a physician were those involving a physician shadowing experience (Clithero et al., 2013).

Some authors stress the importance of including a variety of training components. Bell and Buelow (2014) state that in their program, "the various experiences were all necessary to ensure achievement of student learning outcomes." (This program comprises an online poverty simulation, reflection and discussion, several online and in-class lessons with corresponding quizzes, interprofessional team assignments, a home visit, weekly clinical work with reflective journals, and a final team presentation.) Others presume that the reading assignments in their program may explain why even those students who had volunteered in shelters previously experienced growth during the training (Feen-Calligan, 2008).

Need for Guidance

Students need a certain level of guidance with regard to their experiential learning. In one of the programs, students suggested the need to provide more hands-on guidance in planning and implementing the community-based projects (O'Brien et al., 2014). Some papers mention the students' initial discomfort with having no predetermined protocols (Feen-Calligan, 2008) or their wish for more structure or a guidebook (Dharamsi et al., 2010a). Nonetheless, some students reported that the lack of predetermined protocols helped them really listen to the children with whom they were working (Feen-Calligan, 2008). Other authors even warn that caution is necessary with respect to the information that is provided about the issues a community faces, as this can sometimes lead to forming biases and stereotyping (Kelly, 2013).

Care for the Students

Some of the papers note explicit attention to the students' well-being. Consideration of students' well-being is evoked by Kelly (2013, p. 35), who mentions that "students are generally more comfortable working in pairs, and pairing students together fosters teamwork, confidence, and safety at service-learning sites." Other authors focus on the fact that the training helped the students protect and foster their idealism (Bakshi et al., 2015) and kept them from becoming cynical (Bakshi et al., 2015; Meili et al., 2011). This was especially the case in elective programs in which the most motivated students were selected to participate.

Nonstudent Evaluations

Almost all papers address the students' point of view, whereas the point of view of trainers or community members is rarely considered. However, Matejic and colleagues (2012) conducted a quantitative evaluation study involving 1,188 students, 630 patients, and 78 physicians. Remarkably, in this study, patients appeared to be more satisfied with the program than were the students and physicians. Mudarikwa and colleagues (2010) also included the perspective of community educators, who valued the students' presence and reported some difficulties related to the project. Also of note is that none of the included studies examined the effect of the program on the community's health.

Cost of the Programs

Most papers include no information on the costs of the program. Occasionally, some information is provided about the size of the workforce required for a program (e.g., Art et al., 2008). O'Brien and colleagues (2014) report that funding constraints limited the number of students that could participate. Some papers mention grants that were available for participating students, mostly to take part in international programs (e.g., Larson et al., 2010; Meili et al., 2011), and occasionally to attend external advocacy skill-building workshops and seminars (Bakshi et al., 2015). In some other cases, program funding was obtained (e.g., Meurer et al., 2011; Sabo et al., 2015).

Difficulties and Bottlenecks

Despite principally positive evaluations, some papers give voice to critical views and describe the difficulties encountered during the program rollout.

Programs often require an enormous amount of time and energy from both the university and the community (Art et al., 2008; Ezeonwu et al., 2014; Kelly, 2013; Sabo et al., 2015). O'Brien and colleagues (2014) state that there is a need to provide salary support to allow faculty and community leaders the time for student guidance. Another program (Sabo et al., 2015) engaged doctoral students as co-instructors with the aim of bringing new energy, directions, and partnerships to the course and helping to alleviate potential burnout among faculty and partners. Other logistic difficulties concern, for instance, placement logistics and contextualization of didactic material at community sites (Mudarikwa et al., 2010). Moreover, students working in the community the same day every week was not considered the ideal way to give them insight into day-to-day life in the community (Mudarikwa et al., 2010). Loss of information and continuity as successive student cohorts transitioned in and out of longitudinal projects was also reported (Bakshi et al., 2015).

Some of the papers mention concerns about students' safety. This was the case, for example, in a program in which students made home visits (Bell and Buelow, 2014). Being accompanied by another student, providing the address and vehicle information to the course faculty, and calling when the visit ended were some of the measures taken to guarantee their safety.

Some authors encountered difficulty in convincing students to participate in the program (Dharamsi et al., 2010b) or to having them keep a reflective journal, although they gradually came to appreciate the latter (Dharamsi et al., 2010b).

CONCLUSIONS AND DISCUSSION

The purpose of this study was to obtain an overview of education programs addressing the social determinants of health in and with communities by searching the literature published on this topic. After strict inclusion criteria were applied to the papers in the original database, 33 papers were selected for this review. As mentioned earlier, we found that fewer papers mentioned "social determinants of health" as a goal (n = 9) than mentioned "health inequity" or "health disparity" (n = 11). Unfortunately, "health inequity" and "health disparity" were not included in the search terms. Thus, relevant papers may have been missed. Moreover, time constraints did not allow us to complete this database with screenings of reference lists or with searches for additional information on the Internet (gray literature and possibly relevant websites[5]). A systematic screening of relevant conference abstract books also was not possible.

The large majority of the programs reviewed (n = 24) are based in the

---

[5] For example, the websites of Community-Campus Partnerships for Health, https://ccph.memberclicks.net/service-learning (accessed January 15, 2016); Training for Health Equity Network, http://thenetcommunity.org (accessed January 15, 2016); or The Network: Towards Unity for Health, http://www.the-networktufh.org (accessed January 28, 2016).

United States and are focused on medicine (n = 10) and/or nursing students (n = 8). Some programs are *obligatory* for all students, while others are *elective or extracurricular*, sometimes available only to selected students. The reasons for allowing only selected students are often not mentioned. Logistic and financial reasons may play a role (Kassam et al., 2013; Meili et al., 2011), as well as ethical reasons (e.g., excluding faculty and students who would participate for personal reasons, thereby harming the community) (Dharamsi et al., 2010b). The particular selection criteria often concern previous experiences, motivations, professional goals, language skills, and quality of reflection and writing (Bakshi et al., 2015; Dharamsi et al., 2010b; Meili et al., 2011), which means that students who are sensitive to the broader social picture often are selected for the programs. The information obtained from the included papers does not allow us to make statements about the impact of a program's being mandatory or not.

The programs reviewed varied greatly in the length and intensity of the training. Nevertheless, a lack of information often prevented us from getting a clear idea of the amount of time the students spent on each of the program components. Moreover, it was often difficult to conclude whether the programs were integrated in a set of study modules or isolated. Moreover, based on the available information, it was not possible to determine whether it is better to have intense immersion experiences or to distribute the time spent in the communities over a more extended period of time. Examples of both were found among the included papers.

Different types of communities are involved in the programs reviewed. Most often they are located in the same region as the schools, but some schools have partnerships with communities farther away or even abroad. When international learning experiences, additional aspects, such as financial support, logistics, and language barriers, need to be considered. One program (Meili et al., 2011) offered the students a broad range of experiences (including 6 weeks in a rural remote community, two shifts per month in an urban student-run clinic, and 6 weeks in a rural hospital abroad).

Service learning was found to be the most commonly used educational approach. Several authors emphasize its different components, which basically encompass both elements of the term "service learning." "Service" refers to the fact that a genuine collaboration with the community should be established. Community members should be involved at all stages of the training and should also benefit from the cooperation. It is an ethical obligation to focus on reciprocal benefits and to avoid the risk of students being involved in "social sightseeing" (Art et al., 2008). Examples of community benefits include direct help from community projects or support through advocacy for the community (e.g., students writing a letter to the editor [Dharamsi et al., 2010a] or presenting survey findings to local key decision makers [Clithero et al., 2013]). In addition, Dharamsi and colleagues

(2010a) stress taking a "social justice" approach and not a "charity" approach. This means that the focus should be not on providing direct service to the community members but on understanding and working to change the structural and institutional factors that contribute to health inequities. Therefore, the sustainability of the campus-community partnership is important. In one of the programs (Kruger et al., 2010), the organizers chose to bolster what the community was already doing "rather than to carve out a niche to address unmet needs and risk competing for scarce resources." The "learning" component of service learning requires not just having students go into to the communities, but stimulating genuine learning among them. This encompasses defining learning goals from the outset, properly preparing students for the learning experience, and guiding them during the community experience. Moreover, reflection is an indispensable component of the training.

Many programs offered a mix of experiential and nonexperiential program components. Experiential learning components included, for instance, conducting community (health) needs assessment, developing and implementing a project or intervention, organizing educational sessions for community members, and caring for individual patients. Nonexperiential learning components included lectures, group discussions, workshops to build capacities, simulation experiences, reading assignments, online activities, presentations, and research projects. Generally, students valued the experiential component highly.

While service-learning experiences appear to be highly valued by educators and students, their effectiveness remains unclear. This observation is in line with the conclusions of Stallwood and Groh (2011) in their systematic review of the evidence on service learning in nursing education. The program evaluation and outcome measurements that are discussed in the present study are generally rather weak and involve considerable risk of various types of biases (e.g., based mainly on self-report, selection of students participating in the program, low numbers of participants, the Hawthorne effect, use of nonvalidated instruments). Moreover, very few papers take the community's perspective into account and none assess long-term effects.

The papers rarely address recruitment of minority students for the programs. Among the included papers, only Parks and colleagues (2015) addressed this issue by establishing a program at four historically black colleges and universities. Although reflecting a slightly different issue, Clithero and colleagues (2013) report selecting a diverse group of high school seniors who were committed to practicing in New Mexico's communities of greatest need.

Whether the programs reviewed could easily be replicated is difficult to answer. In many papers, crucial information needed to answer this question is lacking (this may be related partly to the word count restrictions journals impose on authors). Nevertheless, several papers offer insight into the most important training components, and a few also describe the difficulties encountered (which may be valuable for future program development).

RECOMMENDATIONS

Based on this review, the following recommendations can be put forward:

1. **With regard to the present study**
   - A further search for other papers to complete this study is needed. Additionally, contacting the authors of some of the most promising programs might be worthwhile.

2. **With regard to further development of this type of learning**
   - Although available information is very limited, overall evaluation of the programs tends to be positive (especially based on qualitative data). This implies that there are arguments to be made for encouraging/favoring further promotion and implementation of these programs.
   - Both components of "service learning" should be carefully incorporated into the training.
   - An appropriate amount of student guidance should be offered. A good balance is necessary between providing information and guidance on the one hand and allowing for student autonomy and confrontations with real-life conditions on the other.
   - Recommendations with regard to the ideal length of training are difficult to make based on the findings of this review. Nevertheless, experiences that are too brief may compromise the reciprocity of the benefits for students and the communities.
   - As time constraints are often mentioned among the difficulties encountered, appropriate measures for dealing with this issue should be taken into account, where possible.

3. **With regard to future research**
   - When introducing a new program, a well-considered evaluation protocol relying on solid research methods should be considered from the beginning.
   - Efforts should be made to publish the results of this research, as they may inspire other authors. Detailed descriptions of the programs (including the difficulties that were encountered in establishing the program) are recommended.
   - Valid and reliable evaluation instruments should be developed.

- All parties (students, trainers, and community members) should be involved in the evaluation process.
- Efforts to obtain data on outcomes and long-term effects should be encouraged. Questions of interest include Is there an impact of the program on students' career choices? Is there an impact on the social determinants of health and on the community's status? Do programs contribute to increased social accountability of institutions for health professional education? and How does the program affect the community's health?

4. **With regard to ethical considerations**
   - As vulnerable populations are directly involved in this type of education, ethical considerations are extremely important. They include, for instance, being careful not to reinforce power relations, as may be the case when upper-class students come to help minority populations. Solid support and preparation by experienced, ethically, and culturally sensitive persons, preferably both at the university and in the community, is recommended.
   - Sustainability of the collaborations should be carefully considered. Interprofessional and intersectoral approaches may be most effective way to stimulate a sustainable community health impact.

ANNEX A-1[6]: SELF-DESIGNED SCREENING TOOL

EVALUATION PAPERS IOM STUDY   Paper (Number, Author, Year)

....

TYPE OF PAPER

Type	Full paper - Conference abstract -
Content	Research - Only descriptive -

PROGRAM

Name of school	
Location of school	
Name of program	
Location of training (which community)	
Duration of training: Total	
Duration of training: Community learning part	
Program in curriculum	Obligatory / Elective / Extracurricular
Participants: Level	Undergraduate students / Postgraduate students / Professionals
Participants: Type of health profession	
Participants: Number	
Start of program	

Described Goal of Training

Educational approach	
Framework/model	
SDH explicit aim	Yes / No
Focus on SDH	Central / Marginal
References to SDH	
SDH discussed as outcome	

---

[6] Part of this Annex A-1, Table A-1, a literature review summary, is available at http://www.nap.edu/catalog/21923.

Content of Training (Components)

IF RESEARCH PAPER

Type	Quantitative / Qualitative / Mixed
Data	
Research topic	
Number of participants	
Main findings (if relevant and not in IOM questions)	
Strength of study - limitations	

IOM QUESTIONS

Was education goal obtained?	
Was the program successful?	
Were there any difficulties?	
Might the training be replicated?	
Any information about the cost?	
Are there any anecdotes that may be included?	
Suggestions formulated by authors	

REFERENCES TO BE CHECKED: Yes / No

ESTEEMED VALUE FOR PRESENT STUDY:

REMARKS:

REFERENCES

Art, B., L. De Roo, S. Willems, and J. De Maeseneer. 2008. An interdisciplinary community diagnosis experience in an undergraduate medical curriculum: Development at Ghent University. *Academic Medicine* 83(7):657-683.

Bakshi, S., A. James, M. O. Hennelly, R. Karani, A. G. Palermo, A. Jakubowski, C. Ciccariello, and H. Atkinson. 2015. The human rights and social justice scholars program: A collaborative model for preclinical training in social medicine. *Annals of Global Health* 81(2):290-297.

Bell, M. L., and J. R. Buelow. 2014. Teaching students to work with vulnerable populations through a patient advocacy course. *Nurse Educator* 39(5):236-240.

Brown, B., P. C. Heaton, and A. Wall. 2007. A service-learning elective to promote enhanced understanding of civic, cultural, and social issues and health disparities in pharmacy. *American Journal of Pharmaceutical Education* 71(1):6-9.

Bussey-Jones, J. C., M. George, S. Schmidt, J. E. Bracey, M. Tejani, and S. D. Livingston. 2014. Welcome to the neighborhood: Teaching the social determinants of health. *Journal of General Internal Medicine* 29:S543-S544.

Clithero, A., R. Sapien, J. Kitzes, S. Kalishman, S. Wayne, B. Solan, L. Wagner, and V. Romero-Leggott. 2013. Unique premedical education experience in public health and equity: Combined BA/MD summer practicum. *Creative Education* 4(7A2):165-170.

De Los Santos, M., C. D. McFarlin, and L. Martin. 2014. Interprofessional education and service learning: A model for the future of health professions education. *Journal of Interprofessional Care* 28(4):374-375.

Dharamsi, S., N. Espinoza, C. Cramer, M. Amin, L. Bainbridge, and G. Poole. 2010a. Nurturing social responsibility through community service-learning: Lessons learned from a pilot project. *Medical Teacher* 32(11):905-911.

Dharamsi, S., M. Richards, D. Louie, D. Murray, A. Berland, M. Whitfield, and I. Scott. 2010b. Enhancing medical students' conceptions of the canmeds health advocate role through international service-learning and critical reflection: A phenomenological study. *Medical Teacher* 32(12):977-982.

Ezeonwu, M., B. Berkowitz, and F. R. Vlasses. 2014. Using an academic-community partnership model and blended learning to advance community health nursing pedagogy. *Public Health Nursing* 31(3):272-280.

Feen-Calligan, H. 2008. Service-learning and art therapy in a homeless shelter. *Arts in Psychotherapy* 35(1):20-33.

Ierardi, F., and E. Goldberg. 2014. Looking back, looking forward: New masters-level creative arts therapists reflect on the professional impact of an interprofessional community health internship. *Arts in Psychotherapy* 41(4):366-374.

Jarrell, K., J. Ozymy, J. Gallagher, D. Hagler, C. Corral, and A. Hagler. 2014. Constructing the foundations for compassionate care: How service-learning affects nursing students' attitudes towards the poor. *Nurse Education in Practice* 14(3):299-303.

Kassam, R., A. Estrada, Y. Huang, B. Bhander, and J. B. Collins. 2013. Addressing cultural competency in pharmacy education through international service learning and community engagement. *Pharmacy* 1(1):16-33.

Kelly, P. J. 2013. A framework for service learning in physician assistant education that fosters cultural competency. *Journal of Physician Assistant Education* 24(2):32-37.

Kruger, B. J., C. Roush, B. J. Olinzock, and K. Bloom. 2010. Engaging nursing students in a long-term relationship with a home-base community. *Journal of Nursing Education* 49(1):10-16.

Larson, K. L., M. Ott, and J. M. Miles. 2010. International cultural immersion: En vivo reflections in cultural competence. *Journal of Cultural Diversity* 17(2):44-50.

Loewenson, K. M., and R. J. Hunt. 2011. Transforming attitudes of nursing students: Evaluating a service-learning experience. *Journal of Nursing Education* 50(6):345-349.

Matejic, B., D. Vukovic, M. S. Milicevic, Z. T. Supic, A. J. Vranes, B. Djikanovic, J. Jankovic, and V. Stambolovic. 2012. Student-centred medical education for the future physicians in the community: An experience from Serbia. *HealthMED* 6(2):517-524.

Meili, R., D. Fuller, and J. Lydiate. 2011. Teaching social accountability by making the links: Qualitative evaluation of student experiences in a service-learning project. *Medical Teacher* 33(8):659-666.

Meurer, L. N., S. A. Young, J. R. Meurer, S. L. Johnson, I. A. Gilbert, S. Diehr, and Urban and Community Health Pathway Planning Council. 2011. The Urban and Community Health Pathway: Preparing socially responsive physicians through community-engaged learning. *American Journal of Preventive Medicine* 41(4):S228-S236.

Mudarikwa, R. S., J. A. McDonnell, S. Whyte, E. Villanueva, R. A. Hill, W. Hart, and D. Nestel. 2010. Community-based practice program in a rural medical school: Benefits and challenges. *Medical Teacher* 32(12):990-996.

O'Brien, M. J., J. M. Garland, K. M. Murphy, S. J. Shuman, R. C. Whitaker, and S. C. Larson. 2014. Training medical students in the social determinants of health: The Health Scholars Program at Puentes de Salud. *Advances in Medical Education and Practice* 5:307-314.

Ogenchuk, M., S. Spurr, and J. Bally. 2014. Caring for kids where they live: Interprofessional collaboration in teaching and learning in school settings. *Nurse Education in Practice* 14(3):293-298.

Parks, M. H., L. H. McClellan, and M. L. McGee. 2015. Health disparity intervention through minority collegiate service learning. *Journal of Health Care for the Poor and Underserved* 26(1):287-292.

Rasmor, M., S. Kooienga, C. Brown, and T. M. Probst. 2014. United States nurse practitioner students' attitudes, perceptions, and beliefs working with the uninsured. *Nurse Education in Practice* 14(6):591-597.

Sabo, S., J. de Zapien, N. Teufel-Shone, C. Rosales, L. Bergsma, and D. Taren. 2015. Service learning: A vehicle for building health equity and eliminating health disparities. *American Journal of Public Health* 105(Suppl. 1):S38-S43.

Schoon, P. M., B. E. Champlin, and R. J. Hunt. 2012. Developing a sustainable foot care clinic in a homeless shelter within an academic–community partnership. *Journal of Nursing Education* 51(12):714-718.

Seifer, S. D. 1998. Service-learning: Community-campus partnerships for health professions education. *Academic Medicine* 73(3):273-277.

Sharma, M.. 2014. Developing an integrated curriculum on the health of marginalized populations: Successes, challenges, and next steps. *Journal of Health Care for the Poor and Underserved* 25(2):663-669.

Sheu, L., C. J. Lai, A. D. Coelho, L. D. Lin, P. Zheng, P. Hom, V. Diaz, and P. S. O'Sullivan. 2012. Impact of student-run clinics on preclinical sociocultural and interprofessional attitudes: A prospective cohort analysis. *Journal of Health Care for the Poor and Underserved* 23(3):1058-1072.

Stallwood, L. G., and C. J. Groh. 2011. Service-learning in the nursing curriculum: Are we at the level of evidence-based practice? *Nursing Education Perspectives* 32(5):297-301.

Stanley, M. J. 2013. Teaching about vulnerable populations: Nursing students' experience in a homeless center. *Journal of Nursing Education* 52(10):585-588.

Ward, S., M. Blair, F. Henton, H. Jackson, T. Landolt, and K. Mattson. 2007. Service-learning across an accelerated curriculum. *Journal of Nursing Education* 46(9):427-430.

Williams, B. C., J. S. Perry, A. J. Haig, P. Mullan, and J. Williams. 2012. Building a curricuum in global and domestic health disparities through a longitudinal mentored leadership training program. *Journal of General Internal Medicine* 27:S552.

Appendix B

Open Session Agenda

Educating Health Professionals to Address the
Social Determinants of Health
A Consensus Study
September 15, 2015
National Academy of Sciences Building
2101 Constitution Avenue, NW
Washington, DC 20418

STATEMENT OF TASK

An ad hoc committee under the auspices of the Institute of Medicine will conduct a study to explore how the education of health professionals is currently addressing the social determinants of health in and with communities. Based on these findings, the committee will develop a framework for how the education of health professionals for better understanding the social determinants of health could be strengthened across the learning continuum.

The committee can consider a variety of perspectives—that could include partnerships, finances and sustainability, experiential learning, continuous professional development, faculty development, policies, systems, and/or health literacy—in preparation of a brief report containing recommendations on how to strengthen health professional education in and with vulnerable communities by addressing the social determinants of health.

OPEN SESSION OF CONSENSUS STUDY COMMITTEE
(webcast event)

SESSION I: ADDRESSING THE SOCIAL DETERMINANTS OF HEALTH

10:00am   **Welcome**
Sandra Lane, Chair of Study Committee

10:15am   **Views of the sponsors**
Moderator: Susan Scrimshaw, Co-Chair, Global Forum on Innovation in Health Professional Education
- Joanna Cain, American College of Obstetricians and Gynecologists/American Board of Obstetrics and Gynecology
- Angelo McClain, National Association of Social Workers
- Shanita Williams, Health Resources and Services Administration
Open microphone for other sponsors' brief remarks

11:15am   **Bringing different sectors together for addressing the social determinants of health**
- Kira Fortune, Advisor on Social Determinants of Health, Pan American Health Organization
Questions and answers

11:45am   **BREAK**

12:00pm   **Presentation of background paper by author**
- Sara Willems, Professor in Health Equity, Ghent University (Belgium via videoconference)
Questions and answers

12:30pm   **LUNCH**

SESSION II: LEARNING BY EXAMPLE

1:30pm **Learning from educational examples**
- The Academy for Academic and Social Enrichment & Leadership Development for Health Equity (Health Equity Academy)
  — Brigit M. Carter, Project Director, Duke University School of Nursing
  Questions and answers
- Florida International University, Herbert Wertheim College of Medicine
  — Pedro J. Greer, Associate Dean for Community Engagement
  — Onelia Lage, Associate Professor, Director of Pediatrics and Adolescent Medicine, Division of Medicine and Society, Department of Humanities, Health, and Society
  — David Brown, Assistant Professor and Chief of the Division of Family Medicine, Department of Humanities, Health, and Society
  Questions and answers

3:00pm **Experiential, community-based learning**
- Medical Education Cooperation with Cuba (MEDICC)
  — Pierre M. LaRamée, Executive Director of MEDICC
  Questions and answers
  — Lillian Holloway, recent graduate of Latin American School of Medicine (ELAM) in Cuba (via videoconference from Cook County Hospital, Chicago)
  Questions and answers
- Challenges and Opportunities of Experiential Learning
  — Elizabeth Doerr, Associate Director of SOURCE (Student Outreach Resource Center), Johns Hopkins University (via videoconference from Baltimore)
  Questions and answers

4:30pm **Open session adjourned**

Appendix C

Global Forum on Innovation in Health Professional Education Sponsors

Academic Collaborative for Integrative Health
Academy of Nutrition and Dietetics
Accreditation Council for Graduate Medical Education
Aetna Foundation
Alliance for Continuing Education in the Health Professions
American Academy of Family Physicians
American Academy of Nursing
American Association of Colleges of Nursing
American Association of Colleges of Osteopathic Medicine
American Association of Colleges of Pharmacy
American Board of Family Medicine
American Board of Internal Medicine
American College of Nurse-Midwives
American College of Obstetricians and Gynecologists/American Board of
    Obstetrics and Gynecology
American Council of Academic Physical Therapy
American Dental Education Association
American Medical Association
American Occupational Therapy Association
American Psychological Association
American Society for Nutrition
American Speech–Language–Hearing Association
Association of American Medical Colleges
Association of American Veterinary Medical Colleges
Association of Schools and Colleges of Optometry

Association of Schools and Programs of Public Health
Association of Schools of the Allied Health Professions
Council of Academic Programs in Communication Sciences and Disorders
Council on Social Work Education
Ghent University
Health Resources and Services Administration
Jonas Center for Nursing and Veterans Healthcare
Josiah Macy Jr. Foundation
Kaiser Permanente
National Academies of Practice
National Association of Social Workers
National Board for Certified Counselors, Inc. and Affiliates
National Board of Medical Examiners
National League for Nursing
Office of Academic Affiliations—Veterans Health Administration
Organization for Associate Degree Nursing
Physician Assistant Education Association
Robert Wood Johnson Foundation
Society for Simulation in Healthcare
Training for Health Equity Network
Uniformed Services University of the Health Sciences
University of Toronto

Appendix D

Speaker Biographies

David Brown, M.D., is founding chief of family and community medicine and vice chair in the Department of Medicine, Family Medicine and Community Health at the Herbert Wertheim College of Medicine and Florida International University (FIU). He has extensive experience with developing innovative educational, outreach, and service-learning programs. At FIU, he has had a leading role in the development of the signature award winning NeighborhoodHELP interprofessional outreach program and related medical school curricula. As founding Family Medicine Residency program director, he developed, launched, and received accreditation for the first residency program initiated by the Wertheim College of Medicine. He is a member of the FIU team for the Association of American Medical Colleges (AAMC) Core Entrustable Activities for Entering Residency Pilot, with a focus on Interprofessional Collaboration and Entrustment. He was co-founder of the Historic Overtown Public Health Empowerment (HOPE) Collaborative and co-editor of the *Overtown Cookbook*. His research interests include urban health, intercultural competencies, interprofessional collaboration, chronic disease prevention and management, integration of behavioral health, household-centered care, and health professions education. His research bricolage involves phenomenological, ethnographic, epidemiologic educational, mixed, and participatory methods. His work has been published in *Social Science and Medicine, American Journal of Public Health, CES4Health.info, MedEdPORTAL, Medical Teacher, The Qualitative Report, American Journal of Obstetrics and Gynecology,* and the *Southern Medical Journal*.

Joanna M. Cain, M.D., FACOG, grew up in the medically underserved Yakima Indian Reservation, and saw firsthand how difficult it is to meet the needs of rural and underserved women. That experience led to the study of medicine after graduating from the University of Washington. She received her M.D. from Creighton University, her residency in obstetrics and gynecology (Ob/Gyn) at the University of Washington and went on to become the first woman accepted for Fellowship in Gynecologic Oncology at Sloan Kettering Cancer Center. She went on to be the first woman president of the Association of Professors of Gynecology and Obstetrics as well as president of the Council of University Chairs for Ob/Gyn. A recognized national leader in women's health nationally and internationally, she continues to focus her research on prevention strategies for gynecologic cancers, medical ethics and curricular development for women's health. She was appointed the first woman and first American Chair of the International Federation of Gynecology and Obstetrics (FIGO) Ethics Committee which she led for a decade. She has served as professor and chair, as well as the Julie Neupert Stott Director of the Center for Women's Health at Oregon Health & Science University (OHSU) where she led the campaign to fund and build an innovative, multidisciplinary Center for Women's Health which is still setting the standard for national development of women's health. She presently serves as professor and vice chair for faculty development at the University of Massachusetts as well as special consultant in women's health Safety and Quality for the American College of Ob/Gyn and Special Rapporteur for Women's Health at FIGO. In these positions, she is developing the American Congress of Obstetricians and Gynecologists (ACOG) Registry Alliance and registries in women's health, the outpatient certification and education programs for safety and quality in women's health and chairing the FIGO initiatives in global cervical cancer control. She is chairing the World Health Organization (WHO) committee working on the cervical cancer control guidance globally.

Brigit M. Carter, M.S.N., Ph.D., joined the Duke University School of Nursing (DUSON) in 2010 and currently serves as the Accelerated B.S.N. (ABSN) Program chair and teaches pediatrics in the undergraduate curriculum. She earned her B.S.N. at North Carolina Central University (NCCU) in 1998, a master's of science in nursing education from University of North Carolina (UNC) at Greensboro in 2002, and a Ph.D. in nursing from UNC at Chapel Hill in 2009. She continues her clinical practice as a staff nurse in the Duke University Medical Center Intensive Care Nursery, where she has 17 years' experience. She is the project director of the Health Resources and Services Administration (HRSA) Nursing Workforce Diversity grant at DUSON, "The Academy for Academic and Social Enrichment and Leadership Development for Health Equity (The Health Equity Academy)," and is also the academic coordinator for this program. Dr. Carter's experience in nursing education before joining the DUSON faculty included coordinating staff education and development in the Intensive Care Nursery, and teaching positions at both Duke (clinical instructor in labor and delivery for ABSN students) and UNC at Chapel Hill (Teaching Fellow in the UNC School of Nursing). Dr. Carter has 26 years of U.S. Navy service (including 9 on active duty) and is currently serving in the rank of Commander in the U.S. Navy Reserves in the Operational Health Support Unit. She is assigned to Naval Medical Center Portsmouth in the Neonatal Intensive Care Unit.

Elizabeth Doerr, M.A., is the associate director of SOURCE (Student Outreach Resource Center), the community service and service-learning center serving the Johns Hopkins University's (JHU's) Schools of Medicine, Nursing, and Public Health. Previously, she was the coordinator for Leadership & Community Service-Learning, Immersion Experiences at the University of Maryland (UMD), College Park. Ms. Doerr has lived, worked, and traveled extensively in Latin America and Africa. Ms. Doerr's work at SOURCE focuses primarily on training faculty in service-learning pedagogy and institutionalizing service-learning and community engagement within the JHU health professional schools. Ms. Doerr is originally from Washington State and earned her M.A. in international education policy from UMD and her B.A. in rhetoric/media studies and Spanish at Willamette University in Salem, Oregon.

Kira Fortune, Ph.D., M.I.H., M.A., has worked more than 15 years in Africa, Asia, Europe, and Latin America in positions related to public health, gender, and social determinants of health. Dr. Fortune spent 4 years working in the Department of Global Advocacy at The International Planned Parenthood Federation in London and then 3 years with the United Nations Children's Fund (UNICEF) in Dar es Salaam, Tanzania, where she was responsible for the program on Prevention of Mother to Child Transmission of HIV (human immunodeficiency virus). Dr. Fortune has extensive experience working with and within nongovernmental organizations (NGOs), academia, and in intergovernmental organizations focusing on gender mainstreaming, social determinants of health, Health-in-All-Policies, and general public health issues. Prior to moving to Washington, DC, she coordinated The International Health Research Network in Denmark with the objective of translating research evidence into policy. In 2008 she joined the Pan American Health Organization, the regional office of the United Nation's WHO, where she is responsible for the Social Determinants of Health and Health in All Policies. Dr. Fortune holds a master's degree in anthropology, development, and gender as well as a doctorate in Sociology on The Challenge of Gender Mainstreaming for a Contemporary NGO from University of London, England. She also holds a master's degree in international public health from Copenhagen University, Denmark.

Pedro J. Greer, Jr., M.D., is professor of medicine at FIU Herbert Wertheim College of Medicine (HWCOM) in Miami, Florida, the chair of the Department of Medicine, Family Medicine and Community Health, associate dean for Community Engagement. Throughout his career, Dr. Greer has been an advocate for health equity by engaging communities to create effective health and social policies and accessible health care systems. His advocacy began during medical training, when he established Camillus Health Concern, Saint John Bosco, health centers for the homeless, underserved, and undocumented populations in Miami-Dade County, Florida. Dr. Greer was recently honored with the 2014 National Jefferson Award in the category of Greatest Public Service Benefiting the Disadvantaged; the award was founded in 1972 by Jacqueline Kennedy Onassis, Senator Taft, Jr., and Sam Beard and the award is often referred to as the Nobel Prize for public service. Dr. Greer was also recognized with the 2013 Great Floridian Award, in 2009 he was awarded with the Presidential Medal of Freedom honoree, receiving America's highest civilian award, the Presidential Service Award in 1997, and in 1993 was named a MacArthur Fellow ("Genius Grant"). He has also received a Papal Medal and has been Knighted as a Knight of Malta and Saint Gregory the Great. He authored *Waking Up in America,* a book about his experiences, from providing care to homeless persons under bridges in Miami, Florida, to advising U.S. presidents on health care, including Presidents Bush Sr. and Clinton. As founding chair of the Department of Humanities, Health, and Society at HWCOM, Dr. Greer spearheaded a unique medical education curriculum to prepare physicians and other health professionals to address the social determinants that affect health access and outcomes, while simultaneously caring for individuals and communities through household visits and engagement. Taking health care to a household centered model. He currently serves in various capacities for a multitude of national, state, and local organizations. He is a Trustee at the RAND Corporation (America's oldest and largest think tank) and is the current Chair of the Pardee RAND Graduate School Board of Governors, the largest Ph.D.-granting institution for policy analysis. Additionally, Dr. Greer served as chair for the Hispanic Heritage Awards Foundation from 2002 to 2012. He is a member of Alpha Omega Alpha National Medical Honor Society and a fellow in the American College of Physicians and the American College of Gastroenterology. Dr. Greer completed his undergraduate degree at the University of Florida and medical studies at La Universidad Catolica Madre y Maestra in the Dominican Republic. He trained in internal medicine and served as chief resident at the University of Miami Miller School Of Medicine in Miami, Florida. Dr. Greer completed two post-doctoral fellowships—one in hepatology and the second in gastroenterology. He is board certified in medicine and gastroenterology.

Lillian Holloway, M.D., grew up in West Philadelphia. She worked as a certified nursing assistant before deciding to go to medical school. She graduated from the Latin American School of Medicine (ELAM), Havana, Cuba, in 2009. She is currently a resident in Family Practice and an M.P.H. candidate at University of Illinois Hospitals in Chicago.

Onelia Lage, M.D., has 25 years of academic medical experience and is board certified in Adolescent Medicine/Pediatrics. In her current position at FIU Herbert Wertheim College of Medicine, she is an associate professor in the Division of Family Medicine and vice chair for education in the Department of Medicine, Family Medicine and Community Health; Assistant Strand Leader for Medicine and Society; director of Pediatric and Adolescent Health for Green Family Foundation NeighborhoodHELP; and associate director of the community engaged physician course. Dr. Lage has served on the Florida Board of Medicine since 2005 and was elected by her peers to serve as chair in 2010. She was the first Hispanic woman to serve in this position. She has been active in leadership with the National Hispanic Medical Association. Her passion lies in helping young people achieve their ultimate potential and preparing the next generation of physicians with a strong emphasis on compassionate care, humility, and ethical and professional character.

Pierre M. LaRamée, M.A., Ph.D., executive director of Medical Education Cooperation with Cuba (MEDICC), has more than 30 years' experience in NGO programming and administration with overlapping expertise in academic research, policy analysis/advocacy, strategic communications/publishing, and resource development. In his nonprofit career, Dr. LaRamée has also developed strong geographical expertise on Latin American and Caribbean political and social issues. Prior to joining MEDICC, he co-founded Re:Generation Consulting, building on his career at International Planned Parenthood Federation-Western Hemisphere Region, where he oversaw communications, media, and fundraising activities while directing emerging cutting-edge advocacy programs in Latin America and the Caribbean. He came to International Planned Parenthood Federation/Western Hemisphere Region (IPPF/WHR) in 2004 from the Puerto Rican Legal Defense and Education Fund, a Latino civil rights organization, where he served as director of development and executive vice president. He previously served as executive director of the North American Congress on Latin America, a research and publishing organization specializing in U.S.-Latin American Relations, and as assistant professor of sociology and

Latin American studies at St. Lawrence University. He is fluent in French and Spanish and has authored and co-authored numerous articles, book chapters, and reviews. Dr. LaRamée holds a master's in political science from McGill University and a Ph.D. in the sociology of international development from Cornell University.

Angelo McClain, Ph.D., LICSW, is the chief executive officer of the National Association of Social Workers (NASW) and president of the National Association of Social Workers Foundation. NASW is the largest membership organization of professional social workers in America with 140,000 members. NASW promotes the profession of social work and social workers and advocates for sound social policies that improve well-being for individuals, families, and communities. Dr. McClain previously served as Commissioner for the Massachusetts Department of Children and Families for 6 years, a position appointed by Governor Deval Patrick. While there, he oversaw a budget of $850 million and a workforce of 3,500 employees to address reports of abuse and neglect for the state's most vulnerable children, partnering with families to help them better nurture and protect their children.

Susan Scrimshaw, Ph.D., M.A., is currently the president of The Sage Colleges in Troy, New York. Prior to her appointment as president of The Sage Colleges, Dr. Scrimshaw was president of Simmons College in Boston, Massachusetts. She was dean of the School of Public Health, and professor of community health sciences and of anthropology at the University of Illinois at Chicago (UIC) from 1994 through June 2006. Prior to becoming dean at UIC in 1994, she was associate dean of public health and professor of public health and anthropology at the University of California, Los Angeles. Dr. Scrimshaw is a graduate of Barnard College and obtained her M.A. and Ph.D. in anthropology from Columbia University. Her research includes community participatory research methods, addressing health disparities, improving pregnancy outcomes, violence prevention, health literacy, and culturally appropriate delivery of health care. She is a member of the National Academy of Medicine, where she has been elected a member of the governing council and serves on the Committee on Science, Engineering, and Public Policy (COSEPUP), a joint unit of the National Academy of Sciences, the National Academy of Engineering, and the National Academy of Medicine. She is also a fellow of the American Association for the Advancement of Science, the American Anthropological Association, and the Institute of Medicine of Chicago. While in Chicago, Dr. Scrimshaw was an appointed member of the Chicago Board of Health and Illinois State Board of Health. She chaired the Institute of Medicine (IOM) Committee on Communication for Behavior Change in the 21st Century: Improving the Health of Diverse Populations, and served as a member of the IOM Committee on Health Literacy. She is a past president of the board of directors of the U.S.-Mexico Foundation for Science, former chair of the Association of Schools of Public Health, and past president of the Society for Medical Anthropology. Her honors and awards include the Margaret Mead Award, a Hero of Public Health gold medal awarded by President Vicente Fox of Mexico, the UIC Mentor of the Year Award in 2002, and the Chicago Community Clinic Visionary Award in 2005.

Sara Willems, M.A., Ph.D., received a master's in health promotion (1999) and a Ph.D. in medical sciences (2005) from Ghent University (Belgium). Since 2005 she coordinates the research group "Inequity in health and primary health care." In 2011 she was appointed as the first professor in health equity at Ghent University. Her research activities focus on the social gradient in medical health care use, the accessibility of the Belgian health care system, the role of primary health care in tackling health inequity, and the link between social capital and health (inequity). She developed a special interest in the use of qualitative research methods. Dr. Willems is the author of chapters in several books and wrote articles in several peer-reviewed journals. She is (co-)author of several research reports for the federal and local authorities. She is involved in the medical curriculum and in the master program on health promotion at Ghent University where she teaches on social inequity, and health and society. She is also involved in the design and implementation of several community health projects in Ghent and is the chief executive officer of a community health center in one of the deprived areas in Ghent.

Shanita D. Williams, Ph.D., M.P.H., APRN, is chief of the Nursing Education and Practice Branch in the Division of Nursing and Public Health, Bureau of Health Workforce at HRSA. As branch chief, Dr. Williams leads the Division of Nursing and Public Health's investments in two key areas—the Nursing Workforce Diversity (NWD) Program, which supports projects that incorporate the social determinants into evidence-based strategies to increase nursing workforce diversity, and the Nurse Education, Practice, Quality and Retention (NEPQR) Program, which supports interprofessional collaborative practice models that include diverse interprofessional teams composed of nurses and other health professionals. Dr. Williams is a member of the National Academies of Sciences, Engineering, and Medicine's Global Forum on Innovation in Health Professional Education and a member of the National Advisory Committee for the Robert Wood Johnson Foundation's Future of Nursing Scholars Program. She is a family nurse practitioner and social epidemiologist; received her bachelor's and master's degrees in nursing from the University of South Carolina in Columbia; her Ph.D. in nursing from Georgia State University in Atlanta; and an M.P.H. degree from the Johns Hopkins School of Hygiene and Public Health in Baltimore, Maryland. Dr. Williams completed postdoctoral training as a Cancer Prevention Fellow at the National Cancer Institute (NCI) in Bethesda, Maryland, in the Division of Cancer Control and Populations Sciences, Surveillance Research Program. Dr. Williams has received an NCI Fellow's Merit Award and Minority Scholar Awards for Cancer Research from the American Association for Cancer Research (AACR). Dr. Williams is also a National Institute on Minority Health and Health Disparities (NIMHD) Research Scholar.

Appendix E

Committee Member Biographies

Sandra D. Lane, Ph.D., M.P.H. (*Chair*), Laura J. and L. Douglas Meredith Professor of teaching excellence, is a professor of public health and anthropology at Syracuse University and a research professor in the Department of Obstetrics and Gynecology at Upstate Medical University. She received her Ph.D. in medical anthropology from the joint program at the University of California, San Francisco (UCSF), and the University of California, Berkeley (UC Berkeley), and an M.P.H. in epidemiology from UC Berkeley. Her research focuses on the impact of racial, ethnic, and gender disadvantage on maternal, child, and family health in urban areas of the United States and the Middle East. In addition to the Meredith award, she received the Carl F. Wittke Award for Distinguished Undergraduate Teaching and the John S. Diekhoff Award for Distinguished Graduate Teaching, both at Case Western Reserve University. Dr. Lane has developed a model that links the community-participatory analysis of public policy with pedagogy, called CARE (Community Action Research and Education). Her CARE projects include food deserts in Syracuse, lead poisoning in rental property, health of the uninsured, and her current project on neighborhood trauma and gun violence. Her CARE publications since joining the Syracuse University faculty have included as co-authors 5 community members, 10 graduate students, and 11 undergrads. Prior to joining Syracuse University, Dr. Lane was the founding director of Syracuse Healthy Start, an infant mortality prevention program, in Syracuse, New York. With Dr. Richard Aubry she developed an intervention for screening and treating pregnant women for bacterial vaginosis that was associated with a 50 percent reduction in premature births in Syracuse ("Evaluation of Syracuse Healthy Start's program for abnormal flora screening, treatment, and rescreening among pregnant women, Syracuse, New York, 2000-2002," (2011) *Maternal and Child Health Journal*, 15(7):1020-1028.) She led a community-wide health literacy initiative that resulted in a 75 percent reduction of post neonatal deaths among women who had not graduated from high school. ("Parental Literacy and Infant Health: An Evidence-Based Healthy Start Intervention," (2006) *Health Promotion Practice*, 7(1):95-102.) She secured grant funding to support the development of the Onondaga County Child Fatality Review Team and served as a member from 1997-2004. She has also been a consultant to WHO for operational research on tuberculosis, United Nations Population Fund (UNFPA) and UNICEF for Rapid Assessment Procedures, and the Joint Commission on the Accreditation of Healthcare Organizations (JCAHO) for qualitative methods in hospital evaluation. From 1988-1992, she was the Child Survival, Reproductive Health and Population Program Officer, in the Ford Foundation's Cairo, Egypt, field office, with grant-making responsibility for Egypt, Jordan, Lebanon, Sudan, the West Bank and Gaza, and Yemen.

Jorge Delva, Ph.D., M.S.W., a native of Chile, is professor of social work and associate dean, School of Social Work at the University of Michigan. He conducts research focusing on addressing and reducing health disparities and helping improve the lives of low-income and racial and ethnic minority populations. His research began in Honolulu two decades ago where he worked on Substance Abuse and Mental Health Services Administration (SAMHSA)-funded projects aimed at improving the health and mental health of Asian and Pacific Islander children and their families. His more recent state and National Institutes of Health (NIH)-funded projects show his dedication to combating health disparities. His work has served to advance the substance abuse field's understanding of psychosocial-cultural mechanisms associated with substance using behaviors among Hispanic/Latino, African American, and American Indians of lower socioeconomic position in the United States and with disadvantaged populations in Latin America.

Julian Fisher, M.Sc., M.I.H., is an experienced policy advisor specializing in public health and the environment. Work experience in a diverse range of professional environments and geographical locations, covering Antarctica, Europe, Falkland Islands, Saudi Arabia, South Africa, and Tanzania within various sectors and organizations, including international public health policy and advocacy, health profession (federation) management, undergraduate and post-graduate education, both classroom and Web based. Currently based at the Medical School Hannover working in a consultancy cooperation with the World Health Organization (WHO). Dr. Fisher earned his B.D.S. (dentistry) from Birmingham University in 1985, his M.Sc. (HIV/

AIDS) from Stellenbosch University in 2002, and his M.I.H. (international health) from Charite University in 2006.

Bianca Frogner, Ph.D., is an associate professor in the Department of Family Medicine and director of the Center for Health Workforce Studies in the School of Medicine at the University of Washington (UW). Dr. Frogner is an NIH-trained health economist with expertise in health workforce, labor economics, health spending, health insurance coverage and reimbursement, international health systems, and welfare reform. She has published in leading health care journals such as *Health Affairs* and *Health Services Research and Medical Care*. Dr. Frogner has been funded by the National Institute of Mental Health, Centers for Disease Control and Prevention, and Health Resources and Services Administration (HRSA). Prior to joining UW, Dr. Frogner was an assistant professor in the Health Services Management and Leadership Department in the Milken Institute School of Public Health at The George Washington University (GW) from 2009 to 2015. At GW, she was the deputy director of the Health Workforce Research Center. Dr. Frogner completed a post-doctoral fellow at the University of Illinois at Chicago School of Public Health in 2009. Dr. Frogner received her Ph.D. in health economics at the Johns Hopkins Bloomberg School of Public Health in 2008. She received her B.A. at the University of California, Berkeley, in molecular and cell biology in 2001.

Cara V. James, Ph.D., is the director of the Office of Minority Health at the Centers for Medicare & Medicaid Services (CMS). Prior to joining the Office of Minority Health at CMS, Dr. James was the director of the Disparities Policy Project and the director of the Barbara Jordan Health Policy Scholars Program at the Henry J. Kaiser Family Foundation, where she was responsible for addressing a broad array of health and access to care issues for racial and ethnic minorities and other underserved populations, including the potential impact of the Patient Protection and Affordable Care Act, analyses of state-level disparities in health and access to care, and disparities in access to care among individuals living in health professional shortage areas. Prior to joining the staff at Kaiser, she worked at Harvard University and The Picker Institute. Dr. James is a member of the National Academies of Sciences, Engineering, and Medicine's Roundtable on the Promotion of Health Equity and the Elimination of Health Disparities and has served on several Institute of Medicine (IOM) committees, including the Committee on Leading Health Indicators for Healthy People 2020. She has published several peer-reviewed articles and other publications, and was a co-author for one of the background chapters for the IOM report *Unequal Treatment: Confronting Racial and Ethnic Disparities in Health Care*. Dr. James received her Ph.D. in health policy and her A.B. in psychology from Harvard University.

Malual Mabur, M.B.B.S., is a graduate of a medical school in Khartoum, Sudan. He obtained his master's degree in Tropical Medicine and International Health from University of London in the United Kingdom. Dr. Mabur received his post-graduate diploma in Tropical Medicine and Hygiene from the Royal College of Physicians of London. He moved to the United States in 2010 and is preparing to sit for the United States Medical Licensing Exam. He has worked in different fields oversees and within the United States. He currently works as Health Promotion Specialist and Community Health Outreach Worker with the City of Portland, Maine. His work is focused on serving the access and navigation needs of the Arabic speaking communities in Portland. Dr. Mabur's position is funded by an HRSA, Nurse Education, Practice, Quality and Retention (NEPQR) grant administered by the University of New England and also through CHANNELS (Community, Health, Access, Network, Navigate, Education, Leadership, and Service), which aims to improve immigrant and refugee health in Maine through innovations in team-based care.

Laura Magaña Valladares, Ph.D., has a bachelor's degree in education, a master's degree in educational technology, and a Ph.D. in educational administration from Gallaudet University in Washington, DC. She is a certified trainer in the cognitive programs of the Hadassah-Wizo-Canada Research Institute of Israel. Dr. Magaña has more than 30 years dedicated to higher education in public and private universities in Mexico; educational organizations in United States; United Nations programs and nongovernmental organizations in Central America and Europe. Among her multiple positions are the following: Advisers' Coordinator in the Special Education Department of Mexico State; Educational Consultant for UNICEF; Dean of the School of Education University of the Americas; Executive Director of the Mexican-American Institute of Cultural Affairs; Consultant for the International Educational Programs, Denmark Government; General Academic Coordinator, Anahuac University; Educational Consultant, Easter Seals, Michigan, USA; Dean, School of Education and Human Development, La Salle University. She has also been a teacher, trainer, and lecturer in diverse forums in national and foreign universities. For the past 10 years she has been the academic dean of the National Institute of Public Health in Mexico leading the most important educational and technological innovation of the school in its 92 years of existence having a regional impact. Her research interest is in learning environments and the use of technology in education. She is member of the National System of Researchers of Mexico (SNI) and the State System of Researchers (SEI). Dr. Magaña is an active member in community educational organizations such as the Mexican Association for the gifted and talented; The International Net for the Education of the deaf person; board member of the College of Arts and Sciences at Oakland University; Executive board member of Troped; Active member of the International Advisory Committee (IAC) of Public Health Global and President of the Capacity Building Committee Global Evaluation and Monitoring Network for Health (GEMNet), among others.

Spero M. Manson, Ph.D. (Pembina Chippewa), a medical anthropologist and professor of psychiatry, heads the American Indian and Alaska Native Programs at the University of Colorado at Denver and Health Sciences Center. His programs include 9 national centers, totaling $65 million in sponsored activities which entail research, program development, and training among 102 Native communities, spanning rural, reservation, urban, and village settings. Dr. Manson has published 160 articles on the assessment, epidemiology, treatment, and prevention of physical, alcohol, drug, as well as mental health problems in this special population. A member of the National Academy of Medicine (NAM), he has received numerous awards, including three Distinguished Service Awards from the Indian Health Services (IHS) (1985, 1996, 2004), the prestigious Rema Lapouse Mental Health Epidemiology Award from the American Public Health Association (APHA) (1998), two Distinguished Mentor Awards from the Gerontological Society of America (2006, 2007), the Herbert W. Nickens Award from the Association of American Medical Colleges (AAMC) (2006), and the George Foster Award for Excellence from the Society for Medical Anthropology (2006). Dr. Manson received his Ph.D. in anthropology from the University of Minnesota.

Adewale Troutman, M.D., M.P.H., CPH, is professor and associate dean for Health Equity and Community Engagement at the University of South Florida. He has an M.D. from New Jersey Medical School, a master's in public health from Columbia University, master's in Black studies from the State University of New York in Albany, and as of October 2009, board certification from the National Board of Public Health Examiners. He is a residency trained family physician graduating from residency at the Medical University of South Carolina. His career has included clinical emergency medicine, hospital administration, academic, and public health practice. He served as an associate professor in the University of Louisville's School of Public Health and Information Sciences while directing the Metro Louisville Department of Public Health and Wellness. His experience includes special consultancies with WHO in Thailand and Japan, health assessment missions in Angola, Jamaica, and Zaire and training in India and Austria. His commitment to justice has evolved into his nationally recognized efforts to create health equity and the supremacy of the social determinants of health, the founding of the first Center for Health Equity at a local health department and the creation of the Mayors Healthy Hometown Movement.

He is also credited with the passage of one of the strongest antismoking ordinances in the country. Dr. Troutman serves a member or past member of the National Board of Public Health Examiners, the Academy for Health Equity, the Health and Human Services Secretary's Advisory Committee on Health Promotion Disease Prevention Healthy People 2020, the Health and Human Services Secretary's Advisory Committee on Infant Mortality, the Board of Directors of Public Health Law and Policy, the Executive Board of the American Public Health Association the African American Heritage Center, and the National Association of County and City Health Officers.

Antonia M. Villarruel, Ph.D., R.N., FAAN, is professor and the Margaret Bond Simon Dean of Nursing at the University of Pennsylvania School of Nursing. Internationally renowned for her leadership in policy, practice, and research, Dr. Villarruel is a former board member of the American Academy of Nursing (AAN) and was elected to the NAM in 2007. Prior to becoming dean, Dr. Villarruel was a professor, the Nola J. Pender Collegiate Chair and the associate dean for research and global affairs at the University of Michigan School of Nursing. She also held a joint faculty appointment in the School of Public Health and was director of the school's WHO Collaborating Center for Research and Clinical Training in Health Promotion Nursing. She led interdisciplinary and multi-school strategic planning processes to help the University of Michigan integrate the research, education, practice and global missions of the school, the health system and the university. Her efforts to support nursing faculty in developing research programs led to a steady increase in funding from the NIH. Among her national leadership roles, Dr. Villarruel is a former board member of the AAN, a board member of the National Academies of Sciences, Engineering, and Medicine's Board on Population Health and Public Health Practice, and co-chair of the Academies' Roundtable on the Promotion of Health Equity and the Elimination of Health Disparities. She received her Ph.D. in nursing from Wayne State University.

National Academies of Sciences, Engineering, and Medicine Staff

Patricia A. Cuff, M.S., R.D., M.P.H., is a senior program officer for the Board on Global Health within the health and medicine division of the National Academies of Sciences, Engineering, and Medicine. Her primary role is the director of the Global Forum on Innovation in Health Professional Education. She is co-directing the study on clinical trials during the 2014-2015 Ebola outbreak and was the Country Liaison to the Uganda National Academy of Sciences, where she worked for 11 years with African academy staff and members in developing their capacity to provide evidence-based science advice to their governments and to their nations. Prior to her role with the African academies, she was the study director for the Committee on the Options for Overseas Placement of U.S. Health Professionals and with the Board on Neuroscience and Behavioral Health. Ms. Cuff joined the Academies staff to work on the report *Microbial Threats to Health: Emergence, Detection, and Response* under the Board on Global Health. Before coming to Washington, DC, Ms. Cuff worked at St. Luke's-Roosevelt Hospital Center in New York City in the field of HIV-nutrition as a counselor, researcher, and lecturer on topics of adult and pediatric HIV. She received an M.S. in Nutrition and an M.P.H. in Population and Family Health from Columbia University, and performed her undergraduate studies at the University of Connecticut.

Megan M. Perez is a research associate (RA) with the Board on Global Health of the National Academies of Sciences, Engineering, and Medicine. She began her tenure with the Institute of Medicine (IOM) in June 2011 as a senior program assistant, and later a research assistant, for the Forum on Global Violence Prevention. There, she worked on activities related to communications and technology for violence prevention, the contagion of violence, the evidence for violence prevention, and elder abuse and its prevention. In December 2012, Ms. Perez began working for the Global Forum on Innovation in Health Professional Education (HPE). On this project, she works on activities related to HPE, such as interprofessional education and community-engaged HPE. She worked on the IOM report *Measuring the Impact of Interprofessional Education on Collaborative Practice and Patient Outcomes*. Ms. Perez is also a volunteer and volunteer coordinator with the Academies' Job Squad, which works with unemployed or underemployed clients on their resumes, cover letters, and job applications. She graduated in May 2011 from the College of Arts and Sciences at Boston College. She has a B.A. with a major in political science and a minor in faith, peace, and justice.

Bridget Callaghan is a research assistant with the Board on Global Health of the National Academies of Sciences, Engineering, and Medicine, where she works with the Global Forum on Innovation in Health Professional Education (Global Forum). Ms. Callaghan first came to the IOM in January 2015 as a senior program assistant for the Global Forum. In 2014, Ms. Callaghan received her B.S. in Community & Nonprofit Leadership and her B.A. in U.S. history from the University of Wisconsin–Madison. She also received minor degrees in environmental studies and American Indian studies. At Wisconsin, Ms. Callaghan conducted community-based research projects concerning food justice and community nutrition education in collaboration with the Gaylord Nelson Institute for Environmental Studies.

Patrick W. Kelley, M.D., Dr.P.H., joined the Institute of Medicine (IOM) in July 2003 as the director of the Board on Global Health. He has subsequently also been appointed the director of the Board on African Science Academy Development. Dr. Kelley has overseen a portfolio of IOM expert consensus studies and convening activities on subjects as wide ranging as the evaluation of the President's Emergency Plan for AIDS Relief (PEPFAR), the U.S. commitment to global health, sustainable surveillance for zoonotic infections, cardiovascular disease prevention in low- and middle-income countries, interpersonal violence prevention in low- and middle-income countries, and microbial threats to health. He also directs a unique capacity-building effort, the African Science Academy Development Initiative, which over ten years aims to strengthen the capacity of eight African academies to provide independent, evidence-based advice their governments on scientific matters. Prior to joining the Academies Dr. Kelley served in the U.S. Army for more than 23 years as a physician, residency director, epidemiologist, and program manager. In his last U.S. Department of Defense (DoD) position, Dr. Kelley founded and directed the DoD Global Emerging Infections Surveillance and Response System (DoD-GEIS). This responsibility entailed managing surveillance and capacity-building partnerships with numerous elements of the federal government and with health ministries in more than 45 developing countries. He also founded the DoD Accession Medical Standards Analysis and Research Activity. Dr. Kelley is an experienced communicator, having lectured in English or Spanish in more than 20 countries. He has published more than 70 scholarly papers, book chapters, and monographs. Dr. Kelley obtained his M.D. from the University of Virginia and his Dr.P.H. in epidemiology from the Johns Hopkins School of Hygiene and Public Health. He is also board certified in Preventive Medicine and Public Health.